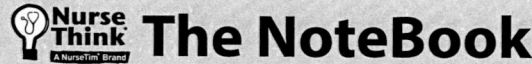

NurseThink® for Students
The NoteBook
Note Taking That Works!
3rd Edition

Tim Bristol, PhD, RN, CNE, ANEF, FAAN
Faculty - Walden University
Minneapolis, Minnesota

Karin J. Sherrill, MSN, RN, CNE, ANEF, FAADN
Faculty - Maricopa Community Colleges
Phoenix, Arizona

NurseThink.com
NurseThink.com/adopt
NurseThink.com/samples

Follow us on Facebook and Instagram!

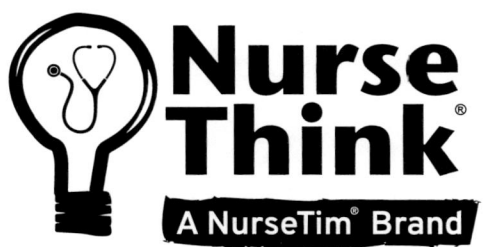

Additional copies of this publication are available at www.NurseThink.com.

ISBN 978-0-9987347-6-7

Printed in the United States of America
Third Edition
0 9 8 7 6 5 4 3 2 1

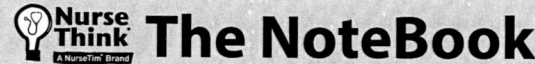
Learning how to learn is essential to the success of every nursing student. Since it is impossible to remember every fact, a clear and consistent process for managing information helps the student develop a deep understanding that applies in any clinical situation. *NurseThink® for Students: The NoteBook* is an easy-to-manage tool that applies clinical judgment when learning course content. This unique tool is ideal for class, reading, studying, collaboration, and even lab and clinical preparation.

As a student begins using the *NurseThink® NoteBook*, they will use clinical judgment skills to prioritize information that is essential to obtain the desired client outcomes. Through a carefully designed process of application and analysis, long-term retention and, more importantly, the ability to adjust to a variety of situations, students create a habit of clinical judgment.

Finally, the *NurseThink® NoteBook* saves students and faculty time and energy. Having concepts visibly organized and quickly accessible allow for better outcomes. Time-savings is a necessity, and this system allows for more focused study.

STUDENT TIPS FOR SUCCESS

Best Practice Study Tips
- While completing your reading, homework, and classroom activities, you will be organizing information in your *NurseThink® NoteBook*.
- Attend and actively engage in class. The classroom facilitator will offer some direction as to where to focus your study. After class (within 24 hours for best success) summarize your classroom discussions in your *NurseThink® NoteBook*.
- Remember you only can choose 3 priorities in each area, so select wisely.

Strategies for Prioritization Power
- Airway, breathing, circulation.
- Maslow's hierarchy; physiologic needs first.
- Determine which findings/potential complications will lead to the greatest chance of mortality or morbidity.
- Identify least invasive interventions first.
- Always consider safety.
- Use the nursing process to identify priorities (assessment, planning, implementation, evaluation).
- Encourage and support self-care with your patient.

Next Gen Learning – NCLEX® Test Plan
These categories are the emphasized areas of your licensure exam. It is important that you become familiar with them so you can best understand what is expected of you on the licensure exam. To see the details of each category, explore the Test Blueprint for the licensure exam you will be taking. (www.ncsbn.org)

Quality and Safety Competencies
National care and safety standards guide our practice. Becoming familiar and applying each of these standards will best prepare you for practice. Consider the situation for your patient with each condition and what emphasis needs to be placed in providing quality care and safety. (www.qsen.org) (www.jointcommission.org)

NurseThink® for Students: The NoteBook tutorials, videos, and additional resources are available at NurseThink.com. If you ever need help with your NurseThink® NoteBook, email help@ nursethink.com.

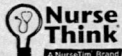
Related Concepts

What Concepts do you need to know about to care for this client? Adaptation? Client preference and profile? Cognition? Comfort? Emotion? Protection? Regulation? Sexuality? Safety Procedures? Check out the index for ideas of related Concepts! When you approach this client—what Concepts come to mind? What concerns you? What care is needed?

Related Exemplars/Diseases

What other Exemplars should I review in my NoteBook? What other Diseases does my client have/is at risk for? What Exemplars/Diseases often accompany this client's chief issues? Consider Crisis, Culture, Health Promotion, Spirituality, Sexuality, Oxygenation? Family Dynamics? Grief? Fluid Imbalance? Nervous system disorders? Pain? Skin? Safety?

Reading/Resources – Clinical Judgment

Go to your readings/Class preparation materials/exercises-What information would you need from the readings to take care of your client?
- What is the pathophysiology of this Exemplar/ Disease?
- How would a client with this Exemplar/Disease look?
- What signs and symptoms are common or particularly troublesome?
- What associated signs and symptoms might you see that occur early in the experience with the Exemplar/ Disease? What might you see late in the experience with the Exemplar/Disease?
- What are the NURSING IMPLICATIONS in the care of clients with this Exemplar/Disease?
- What equipment will you need to care for a client with this Exemplar/Disease?
- What precautions or isolation procedures are needed in the care of a client with this Exemplar/ Disease?

Class/Lab/Clinical – Clinical Judgment

Class/Lab/Clinical
- Your Instructor will provide you with more material in Class/Lab/Clinical.
- What are the general priorities of care when caring for a client with this disease/exemplar?
- Pair up with a peer and compare your notes on the left—what is the same/different-Use Compare and Contrast to REALLY think about The NoteBook page.
- Instructor or Peer: Share experiences of the care of clients with this Exemplar/Disease.
- Refer to the questions/areas on the left to supplement your Class/Clinical/Lab information?
- Create a small group and discuss what you wrote and how The NoteBook additions are the same/different. Supplement your notes.
- Consider your client's care throughout these activities.
- Following a rich discussion of these notes, complete your priorities of care below.

Priority Assessments or Cues

1. What are the three most common assessment/data collection findings or cues that something is different?
2. Write in pencil, priority cues may change, or new information may show up!
3. How would this client look? How would you assess or collect data on the client? How do these alter with changes in status?

Priority Labs & Diagnostics

1. What labs and diagnostics would you need to plan care for this client? What critical values do you need to know?
2. What diagnostic/lab findings would guide the plan of care?
3. How should the nurse care for the client having these labs and diagnostics? What client teaching/preparation is needed?

Priority Nursing Interventions

1. What intervention needs to be done first? What intervention/action can be done fast? How would you know if they worked?
2. What additional actions are needed? What can be delegated/assigned?
3. What equipment do you need? What isolation precautions are needed? What client teaching is needed for precautions?

Priority Medications

1. What medications are critical for this client? What healthcare provider prescriptions are needed?
2. What therapeutic and side effects should be observed? Adverse reactions?
3. What client education is indicated with each medication? What nursing implications guide medication administration?

Priority Potential & Actual Complications

1. What complications could occur if the nurse did not intervene? What interventions are critical to prevent complications?
2. How do these complications guide the plan of care and nursing interventions?
3. What client education/discharge education is needed to prevent potential complications/ address actual complications?

Priority Collaborative Goals

1. What client goals direct your nursing care and interventions? What client teaching/ reinforcement of teaching is indicated?
2. What other members of the healthcare team will assist you in meeting these goals?
3. What care can be delegated/assigned to unlicensed assistive personnel? What care must be done by an RN? An LPN?

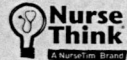
NurseThink® Quick

Pathophysiology-more detail	Pharmacology-more detail	Create a Concept Map
Create a plan of care	Write a test item	Mnemonics
Create a teaching plan	Medication list	Multidisciplinary plan of care
Discharge priorities/Home-based care	Space for additional notes	Clarity the "muddiest part"
Compare and Contrast	Quick Write	Your memory strategies
Ah-Ha's-what you didn't know about or think about before	• Ask 3 questions-Why?	Hints from peers and faculty
	• E3 – Expand Every Event	Study plan

NEXT GEN LEARNING – NCLEX® TEST PLAN

Safe and Effective Care (Management of Care, Coordinated Care, Safety and Infection Control): Threats to safety, Prevention of illness, accidents, and injury, Working with other HCP, Delegation/Assignment, Priorities of care, Leadership principles, Multidisciplinary team, Clients' rights/Informed consent, Advance directives, Case Management, Incidence/variance reports, Dealing with conflict, Change theory, Standard and transmission based precautions, Home safety, Restraints, Safe use of equipment, Disposal of medications/hazardous waste,

Health Promotion and Maintenance: Health assessment, Health promotion, Developmental stages, Impact of growth and development on care, Issues with Aging/Older adults, Screening/immunizations, Lifestyle choices/Risk reduction, Client education, Prevention/wellness

Psychosocial Integrity: Dealing with stress/crisis, Coping, Grief/bereavement/loss, Persistent/significant mental pathology, Psychotropic medications, Therapeutic environment, Therapeutic communication, Abuse, End-of-life concepts, Cultural awareness, Mental health

Physiological Integrity (Basic Care and Comfort, Pharmacological and Parenteral Therapies, Reduction of Risk Potential, and Physiological Adaptation): Daily and therapeutic nutrition, Administering Medications, Skills and procedures, Prevention of Complications, Assessing therapeutic and side effects of medications, Administering fluids/IV therapy, Disease processes/signs/symptoms

QUALITY AND SAFETY COMPETENCIES

Patient-Centered Care: What measures keep the client at the center of the care? What are client and family priorities? Informed consent, Family-centered practices, Implications of family care, Post-discharge issues, Home care, Family dynamics, Client education, Evaluation of learning, Patient-centered versus nurse/agency-centered policies and practices, Respect for self-care

Teamwork and Collaboration: Documentation, Hand-Off report, SBAR, Professional Communication, Relationships, Conflict resolution, Working in groups/group dynamics, Shared decision-making, Mutual respect, Lateral violence, Workplace violence, Community concepts

Evidence-Based Practice: Ensuring best practices, Current practices, New ways to address issues, Standards of care or practice, Delegation of practices, Scope of Practice, Evidence-based skills and procedures, Current research, Trends in care based in evidence

Quality Improvement: Ways to make care more effective, Measurement and evaluation of effectiveness, Communication of quality improvement projects, Focus on outcomes, Quality improvement projects, Participation in quality improvement efforts/initiatives

Safety: Safe medication and parenteral administration, Interventions to keep the client and the nurse safe, Fall, error, and infection prevention, Safe skills and procedures, Infection control measures, Home safety, Limiting exposure to threats to safety

Informatics: Documentation in the Electronic health/medical record, Confidentiality/HIPAA, Telehealth, Patient education, Monitoring/remote monitoring, Infusion devices, Technology, New advances in care, Error prevention, Communication

Peer Review:_____   **Faculty Review:** _____

Grade Tracker:

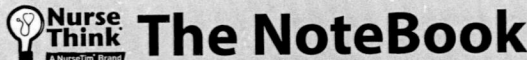
⎯⎧⎯ = *High Frequency Patient Alerts from AARP, AHRQ, CDC and Healthy People 2030* 💡 = *NurseThink® Quick!*

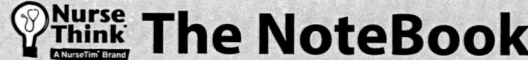
-↓- = High Frequency Patient Alerts from AARP, AHRQ, CDC and Healthy People 2030 💡 *= NurseThink® Quick!*

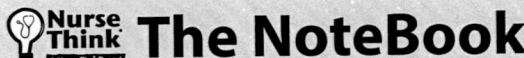
✛ = High Frequency Patient Alerts from AARP, AHRQ, CDC and Healthy People 2030 💡 = NurseThink® Quick!

= High Frequency Patient Alerts from AARP, AHRQ, CDC and Healthy People 2030 = NurseThink® Quick!

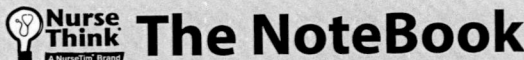

Related Concepts	**Related Exemplars/Diseases**

Reading/Resources - Clinical Judgment	**Class/Lab/Clinical – Clinical Judgment**

Priority Assessments or Cues	**Priority Labs & Diagnostics**	**Priority Nursing Interventions**
1	1	1
2	2	2
3	3	3

Priority Medications	**Priority Potential & Actual Complications**	**Priority Collaborative Goals**
1	1	1
2	2	2
3	3	3

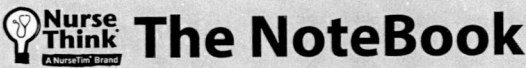
NurseThink® Quick

NEXT GEN LEARNING – NCLEX® TEST PLAN

Safe and Effective Care: Management of Care, Coordinated Care, Safety and Infection Control

Health Promotion and Maintenance

Psychosocial Integrity

Physiological Integrity: Basic Care and Comfort, Pharmacological and Parenteral Therapies, Reduction of Risk Potential, and Physiological Adaptation

QUALITY AND SAFETY COMPETENCIES

Patient-Centered Care

Teamwork and Collaboration

Evidence-Based Practice

Quality Improvement

Safety

Informatics

Peer Review: _____   Faculty Review: _____

Grade Tracker

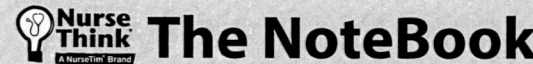
Related Concepts	**Related Exemplars/Diseases**

Reading/Resources - Clinical Judgment	**Class/Lab/Clinical – Clinical Judgment**

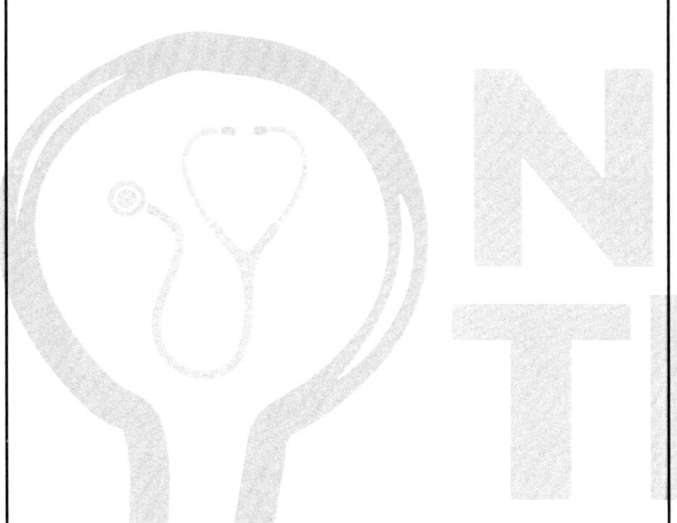

Priority Assessments or Cues	**Priority Labs & Diagnostics**	**Priority Nursing Interventions**
1	1	1
2	2	2
3	3	3

Priority Medications	**Priority Potential & Actual Complications**	**Priority Collaborative Goals**
1	1	1
2	2	2
3	3	3

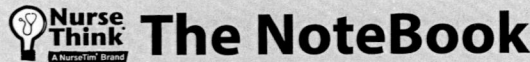
NurseThink® Quick

NEXT GEN LEARNING – NCLEX® TEST PLAN

Safe and Effective Care: Management of Care, Coordinated Care, Safety and Infection Control

Health Promotion and Maintenance

Psychosocial Integrity

Physiological Integrity: Basic Care and Comfort, Pharmacological and Parenteral Therapies, Reduction of Risk Potential, and Physiological Adaptation

QUALITY AND SAFETY COMPETENCIES

Patient-Centered Care

Teamwork and Collaboration

Evidence-Based Practice

Quality Improvement

Safety

Informatics

Peer Review: _____   Faculty Review: _____

Grade Tracker

Related Concepts

Related Exemplars/Diseases

Reading/Resources - Clinical Judgment

Class/Lab/Clinical – Clinical Judgment

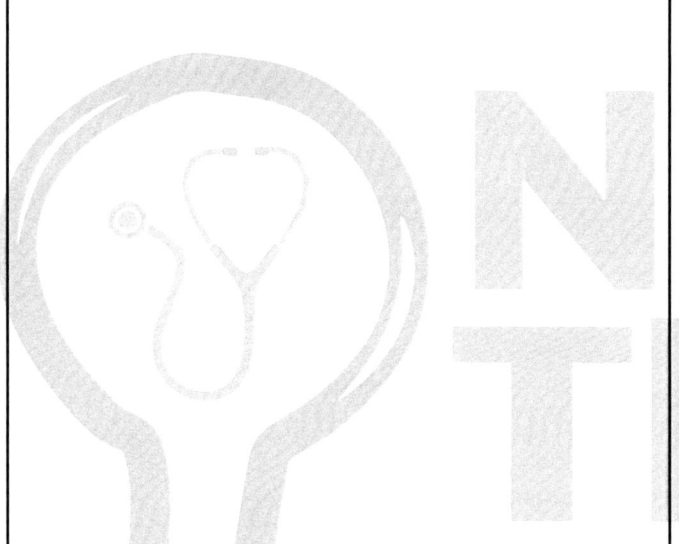

Priority Assessments or Cues

1

2

3

Priority Labs & Diagnostics

1

2

3

Priority Nursing Interventions

1

2

3

Priority Medications

1

2

3

Priority Potential & Actual Complications

1

2

3

Priority Collaborative Goals

1

2

3

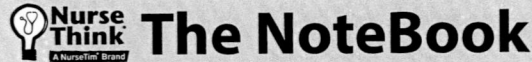
NurseThink® Quick

NEXT GEN LEARNING – NCLEX® TEST PLAN

Safe and Effective Care: Management of Care, Coordinated Care, Safety and Infection Control

Health Promotion and Maintenance

Psychosocial Integrity

Physiological Integrity: Basic Care and Comfort, Pharmacological and Parenteral Therapies, Reduction of Risk Potential, and Physiological Adaptation

QUALITY AND SAFETY COMPETENCIES

Patient-Centered Care

Teamwork and Collaboration

Evidence-Based Practice

Quality Improvement

Safety

Informatics

Peer Review: _____   Faculty Review: _____

Grade Tracker

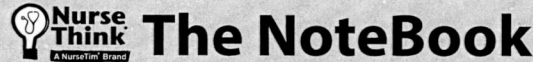

Related Concepts	Related Exemplars/Diseases

Reading/Resources - Clinical Judgment	Class/Lab/Clinical – Clinical Judgment
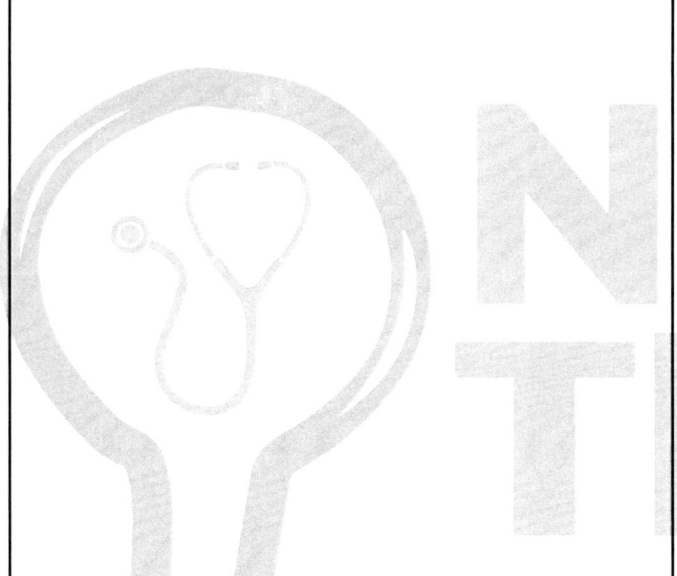	

Priority Assessments or Cues	Priority Labs & Diagnostics	Priority Nursing Interventions
1	1	1
2	2	2
3	3	3

Priority Medications	Priority Potential & Actual Complications	Priority Collaborative Goals
1	1	1
2	2	2
3	3	3

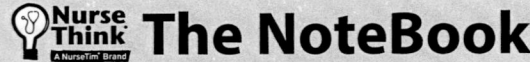
NurseThink® Quick

NEXT GEN LEARNING – NCLEX® TEST PLAN

Safe and Effective Care: Management of Care, Coordinated Care, Safety and Infection Control

Health Promotion and Maintenance

Psychosocial Integrity

Physiological Integrity: Basic Care and Comfort, Pharmacological and Parenteral Therapies, Reduction of Risk Potential, and Physiological Adaptation

QUALITY AND SAFETY COMPETENCIES

Patient-Centered Care

Teamwork and Collaboration

Evidence-Based Practice

Quality Improvement

Safety

Informatics

Peer Review: _____ Faculty Review: _____

Grade Tracker

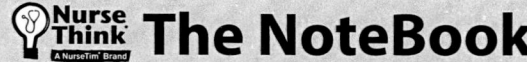
Related Concepts

Related Exemplars/Diseases

Reading/Resources - Clinical Judgment

Class/Lab/Clinical – Clinical Judgment

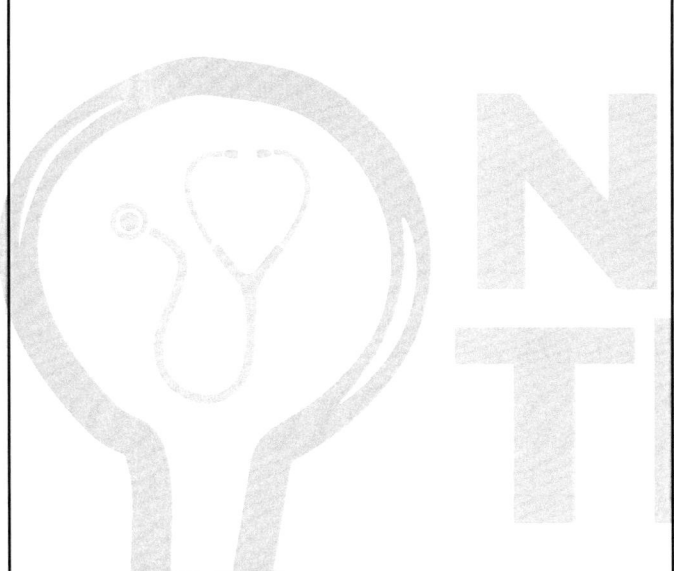

Priority Assessments or Cues

1

2

3

Priority Labs & Diagnostics

1

2

3

Priority Nursing Interventions

1

2

3

Priority Medications

1

2

3

Priority Potential & Actual Complications

1

2

3

Priority Collaborative Goals

1

2

3

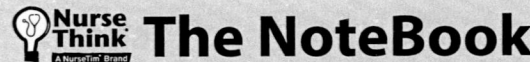
NurseThink® Quick

NEXT GEN LEARNING – NCLEX® TEST PLAN

Safe and Effective Care: Management of Care, Coordinated Care, Safety and Infection Control

Health Promotion and Maintenance

Psychosocial Integrity

Physiological Integrity: Basic Care and Comfort, Pharmacological and Parenteral Therapies, Reduction of Risk Potential, and Physiological Adaptation

QUALITY AND SAFETY COMPETENCIES

Patient-Centered Care

Teamwork and Collaboration

Evidence-Based Practice

Quality Improvement

Safety

Informatics

Peer Review: _____ Faculty Review: _____

Grade Tracker

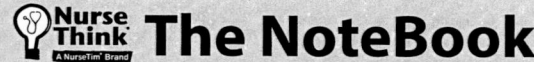
Related Concepts

Related Exemplars/Diseases

Reading/Resources - Clinical Judgment

Class/Lab/Clinical – Clinical Judgment

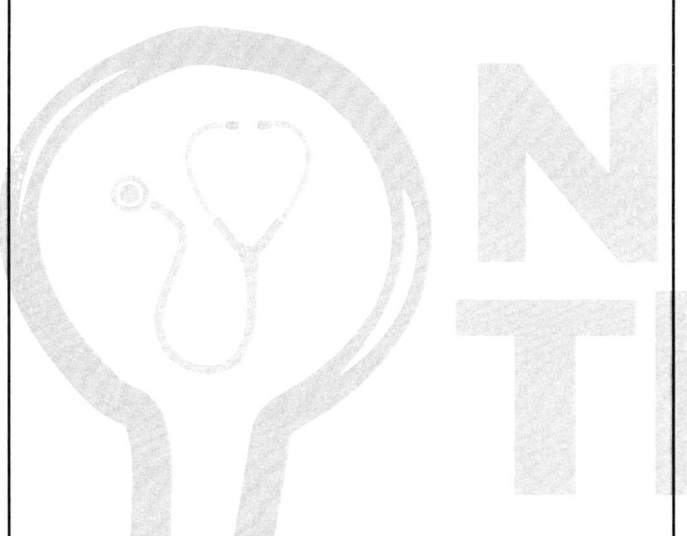

Priority Assessments or Cues

1

2

3

Priority Labs & Diagnostics

1

2

3

Priority Nursing Interventions

1

2

3

Priority Medications

1

2

3

Priority Potential & Actual Complications

1

2

3

Priority Collaborative Goals

1

2

3

The NoteBook

NurseThink® Quick

NEXT GEN LEARNING – NCLEX® TEST PLAN

Safe and Effective Care: Management of Care, Coordinated Care, Safety and Infection Control

Health Promotion and Maintenance

Psychosocial Integrity

Physiological Integrity: Basic Care and Comfort, Pharmacological and Parenteral Therapies, Reduction of Risk Potential, and Physiological Adaptation

QUALITY AND SAFETY COMPETENCIES

Patient-Centered Care

Teamwork and Collaboration

Evidence-Based Practice

Quality Improvement

Safety

Informatics

Peer Review: _____   Faculty Review: _____

Grade Tracker

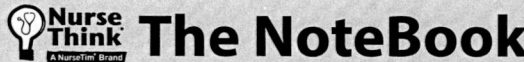
Related Concepts	Related Exemplars/Diseases

Reading/Resources - Clinical Judgment	Class/Lab/Clinical – Clinical Judgment

Priority Assessments or Cues	Priority Labs & Diagnostics	Priority Nursing Interventions
1	1	1
2	2	2
3	3	3

Priority Medications	Priority Potential & Actual Complications	Priority Collaborative Goals
1	1	1
2	2	2
3	3	3

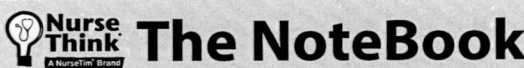
NurseThink® Quick

NEXT GEN LEARNING – NCLEX® TEST PLAN

Safe and Effective Care: Management of Care, Coordinated Care, Safety and Infection Control

Health Promotion and Maintenance

Psychosocial Integrity

Physiological Integrity: Basic Care and Comfort, Pharmacological and Parenteral Therapies, Reduction of Risk Potential, and Physiological Adaptation

QUALITY AND SAFETY COMPETENCIES

Patient-Centered Care

Teamwork and Collaboration

Evidence-Based Practice

Quality Improvement

Safety

Informatics

Peer Review: _____   Faculty Review: _____

Grade Tracker

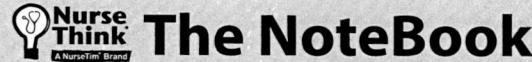
Related Concepts	**Related Exemplars/Diseases**

Reading/Resources - Clinical Judgment	**Class/Lab/Clinical – Clinical Judgment**

Priority Assessments or Cues	**Priority Labs & Diagnostics**	**Priority Nursing Interventions**
1	1	1
2	2	2
3	3	3

Priority Medications	**Priority Potential & Actual Complications**	**Priority Collaborative Goals**
1	1	1
2	2	2
3	3	3

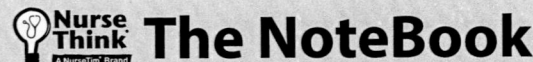
NurseThink® Quick

NEXT GEN LEARNING – NCLEX® TEST PLAN

Safe and Effective Care: Management of Care, Coordinated Care, Safety and Infection Control

Health Promotion and Maintenance

Psychosocial Integrity

Physiological Integrity: Basic Care and Comfort, Pharmacological and Parenteral Therapies, Reduction of Risk Potential, and Physiological Adaptation

QUALITY AND SAFETY COMPETENCIES

Patient-Centered Care

Teamwork and Collaboration

Evidence-Based Practice

Quality Improvement

Safety

Informatics

Peer Review: _____   Faculty Review: _____

Grade Tracker

Related Concepts

Related Exemplars/Diseases

Reading/Resources - Clinical Judgment

Class/Lab/Clinical – Clinical Judgment

Priority Assessments or Cues

1
2
3

Priority Labs & Diagnostics

1
2
3

Priority Nursing Interventions

1
2
3

Priority Medications

1
2
3

Priority Potential & Actual Complications

1
2
3

Priority Collaborative Goals

1
2
3

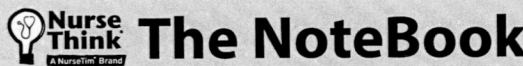

NurseThink® Quick

NEXT GEN LEARNING – NCLEX® TEST PLAN

Safe and Effective Care: Management of Care, Coordinated Care, Safety and Infection Control

Health Promotion and Maintenance

Psychosocial Integrity

Physiological Integrity: Basic Care and Comfort, Pharmacological and Parenteral Therapies, Reduction of Risk Potential, and Physiological Adaptation

QUALITY AND SAFETY COMPETENCIES

Patient-Centered Care

Teamwork and Collaboration

Evidence-Based Practice

Quality Improvement

Safety

Informatics

Peer Review: _____   Faculty Review: _____

Grade Tracker

Related Concepts

Related Exemplars/Diseases

Reading/Resources - Clinical Judgment

Class/Lab/Clinical – Clinical Judgment

Priority Assessments or Cues

1
2
3

Priority Labs & Diagnostics

1
2
3

Priority Nursing Interventions

1
2
3

Priority Medications

1

2

3

Priority Potential & Actual Complications

1

2

3

Priority Collaborative Goals

1

2

3

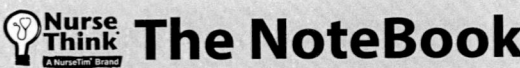
NurseThink® Quick

NEXT GEN LEARNING – NCLEX® TEST PLAN

Safe and Effective Care: Management of Care, Coordinated Care, Safety and Infection Control

Health Promotion and Maintenance

Psychosocial Integrity

Physiological Integrity: Basic Care and Comfort, Pharmacological and Parenteral Therapies, Reduction of Risk Potential, and Physiological Adaptation

QUALITY AND SAFETY COMPETENCIES

Patient-Centered Care

Teamwork and Collaboration

Evidence-Based Practice

Quality Improvement

Safety

Informatics

Peer Review: _____ Faculty Review: _____

Grade Tracker

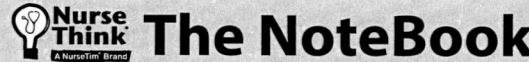

Related Concepts	**Related Exemplars/Diseases**

Reading/Resources - Clinical Judgment	**Class/Lab/Clinical – Clinical Judgment**

Priority Assessments or Cues	**Priority Labs & Diagnostics**	**Priority Nursing Interventions**
1	1	1
2	2	2
3	3	3

Priority Medications	**Priority Potential & Actual Complications**	**Priority Collaborative Goals**
1	1	1
2	2	2
3	3	3

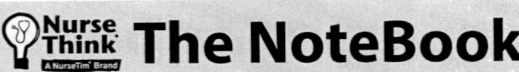
NurseThink® Quick

NEXT GEN LEARNING – NCLEX® TEST PLAN

Safe and Effective Care: Management of Care, Coordinated Care, Safety and Infection Control

Health Promotion and Maintenance

Psychosocial Integrity

Physiological Integrity: Basic Care and Comfort, Pharmacological and Parenteral Therapies, Reduction of Risk Potential, and Physiological Adaptation

QUALITY AND SAFETY COMPETENCIES

Patient-Centered Care

Teamwork and Collaboration

Evidence-Based Practice

Quality Improvement

Safety

Informatics

Peer Review: _____   Faculty Review: _____

Grade Tracker

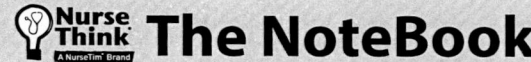
Related Concepts	Related Exemplars/Diseases

Reading/Resources - Clinical Judgment	Class/Lab/Clinical – Clinical Judgment

Priority Assessments or Cues	Priority Labs & Diagnostics	Priority Nursing Interventions
1	1	1
2	2	2
3	3	3

Priority Medications	Priority Potential & Actual Complications	Priority Collaborative Goals
1	1	1
2	2	2
3	3	3

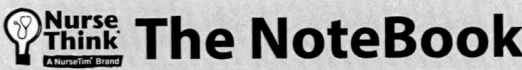
NurseThink® Quick

NEXT GEN LEARNING – NCLEX® TEST PLAN

Safe and Effective Care: Management of Care, Coordinated Care, Safety and Infection Control

Health Promotion and Maintenance

Psychosocial Integrity

Physiological Integrity: Basic Care and Comfort, Pharmacological and Parenteral Therapies, Reduction of Risk Potential, and Physiological Adaptation

QUALITY AND SAFETY COMPETENCIES

Patient-Centered Care

Teamwork and Collaboration

Evidence-Based Practice

Quality Improvement

Safety

Informatics

Peer Review: _____   Faculty Review: _____

Grade Tracker

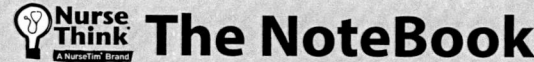
Related Concepts	**Related Exemplars/Diseases**

Reading/Resources - Clinical Judgment	**Class/Lab/Clinical – Clinical Judgment**

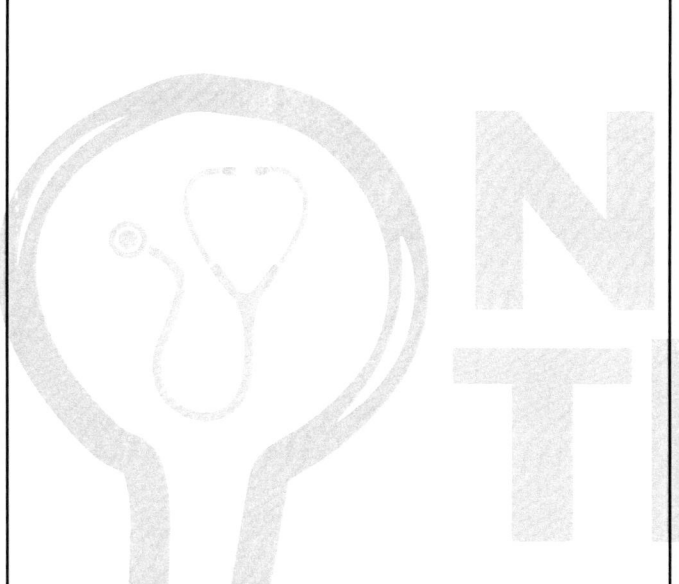

Priority Assessments or Cues	**Priority Labs & Diagnostics**	**Priority Nursing Interventions**
1	1	1
2	2	2
3	3	3

Priority Medications	**Priority Potential & Actual Complications**	**Priority Collaborative Goals**
1	1	1
2	2	2
3	3	3

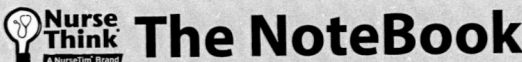

NurseThink® Quick

NEXT GEN LEARNING – NCLEX® TEST PLAN

Safe and Effective Care: Management of Care, Coordinated Care, Safety and Infection Control

Health Promotion and Maintenance

Psychosocial Integrity

Physiological Integrity: Basic Care and Comfort, Pharmacological and Parenteral Therapies, Reduction of Risk Potential, and Physiological Adaptation

QUALITY AND SAFETY COMPETENCIES

Patient-Centered Care

Teamwork and Collaboration

Evidence-Based Practice

Quality Improvement

Safety

Informatics

Peer Review: _____   Faculty Review: _____

Grade Tracker

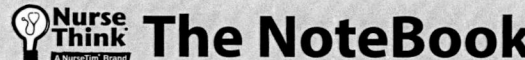

Related Concepts	Related Exemplars/Diseases

Reading/Resources - Clinical Judgment	Class/Lab/Clinical – Clinical Judgment

Priority Assessments or Cues	Priority Labs & Diagnostics	Priority Nursing Interventions
1	1	1
2	2	2
3	3	3

Priority Medications	Priority Potential & Actual Complications	Priority Collaborative Goals
1	1	1
2	2	2
3	3	3

NurseThink® Quick

NEXT GEN LEARNING – NCLEX® TEST PLAN

Safe and Effective Care: Management of Care, Coordinated Care, Safety and Infection Control

Health Promotion and Maintenance

Psychosocial Integrity

Physiological Integrity: Basic Care and Comfort, Pharmacological and Parenteral Therapies, Reduction of Risk Potential, and Physiological Adaptation

QUALITY AND SAFETY COMPETENCIES

Patient-Centered Care

Teamwork and Collaboration

Evidence-Based Practice

Quality Improvement

Safety

Informatics

Peer Review: _____   Faculty Review: _____

Grade Tracker

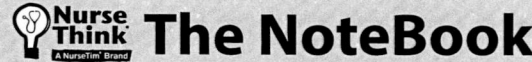

Related Concepts	**Related Exemplars/Diseases**

Reading/Resources - Clinical Judgment	**Class/Lab/Clinical – Clinical Judgment**

Priority Assessments or Cues	**Priority Labs & Diagnostics**	**Priority Nursing Interventions**
1	1	1
2	2	2
3	3	3

Priority Medications	**Priority Potential & Actual Complications**	**Priority Collaborative Goals**
1	1	1
2	2	2
3	3	3

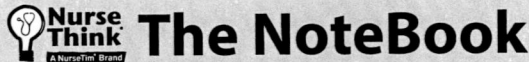

NurseThink® Quick

Nicotinic Effects ***MTWThF*** **M**ydriasis/Muscle cramps **T**achycardia **W**eakness **T**witching **H**ypertension/Hyperglycemia **F**asciculation		

NEXT GEN LEARNING – NCLEX® TEST PLAN

Safe and Effective Care: Management of Care, Coordinated Care, Safety and Infection Control

Health Promotion and Maintenance

Psychosocial Integrity

Physiological Integrity: Basic Care and Comfort, Pharmacological and Parenteral Therapies, Reduction of Risk Potential, and Physiological Adaptation

QUALITY AND SAFETY COMPETENCIES

Patient-Centered Care

Teamwork and Collaboration

Evidence-Based Practice

Quality Improvement

Safety

Informatics

Peer Review: _____   Faculty Review: _____

Grade Tracker

Related Concepts

Related Exemplars/Diseases

Reading/Resources - Clinical Judgment

Class/Lab/Clinical – Clinical Judgment

Priority Assessments or Cues

1
2
3

Priority Labs & Diagnostics

1
2
3

Priority Nursing Interventions

1
2
3

Priority Medications

1

2

3

Priority Potential & Actual Complications

1

2

3

Priority Collaborative Goals

1

2

3

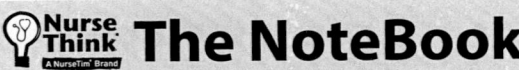

The NoteBook

Prescription Medication Abuse

NurseThink® Quick

NEXT GEN LEARNING – NCLEX® TEST PLAN

Safe and Effective Care: Management of Care, Coordinated Care, Safety and Infection Control

Health Promotion and Maintenance

Psychosocial Integrity

Physiological Integrity: Basic Care and Comfort, Pharmacological and Parenteral Therapies, Reduction of Risk Potential, and Physiological Adaptation

QUALITY AND SAFETY COMPETENCIES

Patient-Centered Care

Teamwork and Collaboration

Evidence-Based Practice

Quality Improvement

Safety

Informatics

Peer Review: _____   Faculty Review: _____

Grade Tracker

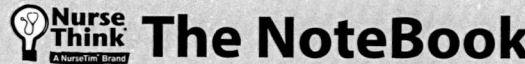

Related Concepts	**Related Exemplars/Diseases**

Reading/Resources - Clinical Judgment	**Class/Lab/Clinical – Clinical Judgment**

Priority Assessments or Cues	**Priority Labs & Diagnostics**	**Priority Nursing Interventions**
1	1	1
2	2	2
3	3	3

Priority Medications	**Priority Potential & Actual Complications**	**Priority Collaborative Goals**
1	1	1
2	2	2
3	3	3

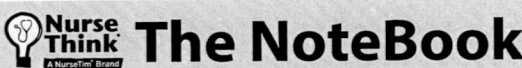

NurseThink® Quick

NEXT GEN LEARNING – NCLEX® TEST PLAN

Safe and Effective Care: Management of Care, Coordinated Care, Safety and Infection Control

Health Promotion and Maintenance

Psychosocial Integrity

Physiological Integrity: Basic Care and Comfort, Pharmacological and Parenteral Therapies, Reduction of Risk Potential, and Physiological Adaptation

QUALITY AND SAFETY COMPETENCIES

Patient-Centered Care

Teamwork and Collaboration

Evidence-Based Practice

Quality Improvement

Safety

Informatics

Peer Review: _____   Faculty Review: _____

Grade Tracker

Related Concepts

Related Exemplars/Diseases

Reading/Resources - Clinical Judgment

Class/Lab/Clinical – Clinical Judgment

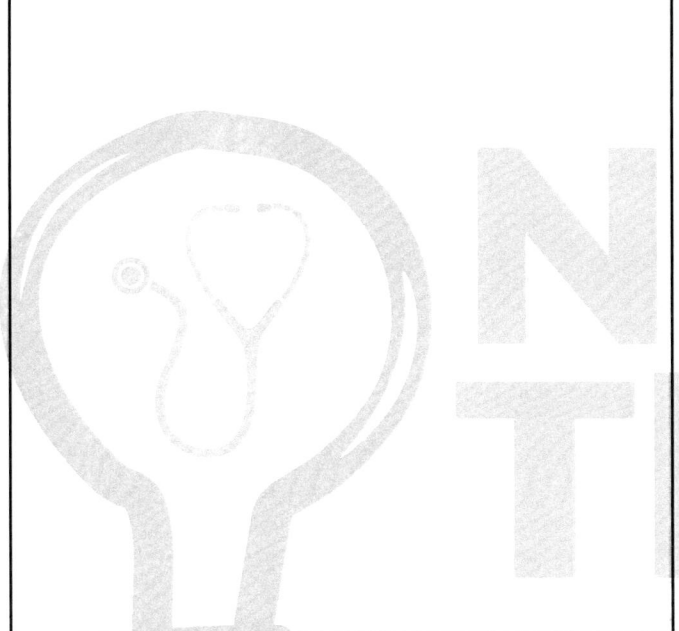

Priority Assessments or Cues	Priority Labs & Diagnostics	Priority Nursing Interventions
1	1	1
2	2	2
3	3	3

Priority Medications	Priority Potential & Actual Complications	Priority Collaborative Goals
1	1	1
2	2	2
3	3	3

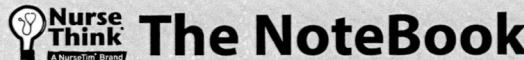
NurseThink® Quick

Abdominal Aortic Aneurism: Symptoms **4A's** **A**symptomatic **A**bdominal mass **A**bdominal pulse **A**ches in low back		

NEXT GEN LEARNING – NCLEX® TEST PLAN

Safe and Effective Care: Management of Care, Coordinated Care, Safety and Infection Control

Health Promotion and Maintenance

Psychosocial Integrity

Physiological Integrity: Basic Care and Comfort, Pharmacological and Parenteral Therapies, Reduction of Risk Potential, and Physiological Adaptation

QUALITY AND SAFETY COMPETENCIES

Patient-Centered Care

Teamwork and Collaboration

Evidence-Based Practice

Quality Improvement

Safety

Informatics

Peer Review: _____   Faculty Review: _____

Grade Tracker

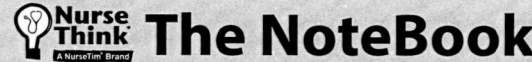
Related Concepts	**Related Exemplars/Diseases**

Reading/Resources - Clinical Judgment	**Class/Lab/Clinical – Clinical Judgment**

Priority Assessments or Cues	**Priority Labs & Diagnostics**	**Priority Nursing Interventions**
1	1	1
2	2	2
3	3	3

Priority Medications	**Priority Potential & Actual Complications**	**Priority Collaborative Goals**
1	1	1
2	2	2
3	3	3

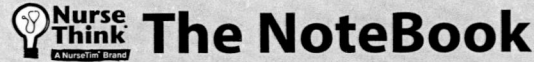
NurseThink® Quick

NEXT GEN LEARNING – NCLEX® TEST PLAN

Safe and Effective Care: Management of Care, Coordinated Care, Safety and Infection Control

Health Promotion and Maintenance

Psychosocial Integrity

Physiological Integrity: Basic Care and Comfort, Pharmacological and Parenteral Therapies, Reduction of Risk Potential, and Physiological Adaptation

QUALITY AND SAFETY COMPETENCIES

Patient-Centered Care

Teamwork and Collaboration

Evidence-Based Practice

Quality Improvement

Safety

Informatics

Peer Review: _____   Faculty Review: _____

Grade Tracker

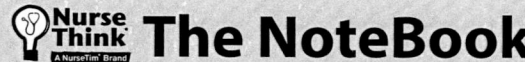

Related Concepts	Related Exemplars/Diseases

Reading/Resources - Clinical Judgment	Class/Lab/Clinical – Clinical Judgment

Priority Assessments or Cues
1
2
3

Priority Labs & Diagnostics
1
2
3

Priority Nursing Interventions
1
2
3

Priority Medications
1
2
3

Priority Potential & Actual Complications
1
2
3

Priority Collaborative Goals
1
2
3

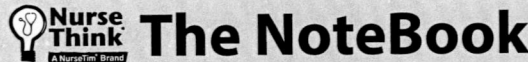
NurseThink® Quick

Raynaud's Phenomenon: Causes	Buerger's Disease Features	
Cold Hand	**Scraps**	
Cryoglobulins/Cryofibrinogens	**S**egmenting thrombosing vasculitis	
Obstruction/Occupational	**C**laudication	
Lupus	**R**aynaud's phenomenon	
Diabetes mellitus/Drugs	**A**ssociated with smoking	
Hematologic problems (polycythemia, leukemia)	**P**ain, even at rest	
Arterial problems (atherosclerosis)	**S**uperficial nodular phlebitis	
Neurologic problems (vascular tone)		
Disease of unknown origin (idiopathic)		

NEXT GEN LEARNING – NCLEX® TEST PLAN

Safe and Effective Care: Management of Care, Coordinated Care, Safety and Infection Control

Health Promotion and Maintenance

Psychosocial Integrity

Physiological Integrity: Basic Care and Comfort, Pharmacological and Parenteral Therapies, Reduction of Risk Potential, and Physiological Adaptation

QUALITY AND SAFETY COMPETENCIES

Patient-Centered Care

Teamwork and Collaboration

Evidence-Based Practice

Quality Improvement

Safety

Informatics

Peer Review: _____   Faculty Review: _____

Grade Tracker

Related Concepts

Related Exemplars/Diseases

Reading/Resources - Clinical Judgment

Class/Lab/Clinical – Clinical Judgment

Priority Assessments or Cues
1
2
3

Priority Labs & Diagnostics
1
2
3

Priority Nursing Interventions
1
2
3

Priority Medications
1

2

3

Priority Potential & Actual Complications
1

2

3

Priority Collaborative Goals
1

2

3

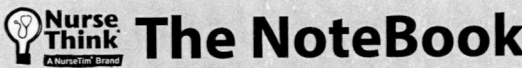
NurseThink® Quick

NEXT GEN LEARNING – NCLEX® TEST PLAN

Safe and Effective Care: Management of Care, Coordinated Care, Safety and Infection Control

Health Promotion and Maintenance

Psychosocial Integrity

Physiological Integrity: Basic Care and Comfort, Pharmacological and Parenteral Therapies, Reduction of Risk Potential, and Physiological Adaptation

QUALITY AND SAFETY COMPETENCIES

Patient-Centered Care

Teamwork and Collaboration

Evidence-Based Practice

Quality Improvement

Safety

Informatics

Peer Review: _____   Faculty Review: _____

Grade Tracker

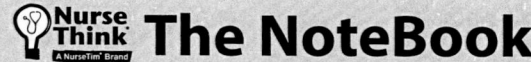
Related Concepts	**Related Exemplars/Diseases**

Reading/Resources - Clinical Judgment	**Class/Lab/Clinical – Clinical Judgment**

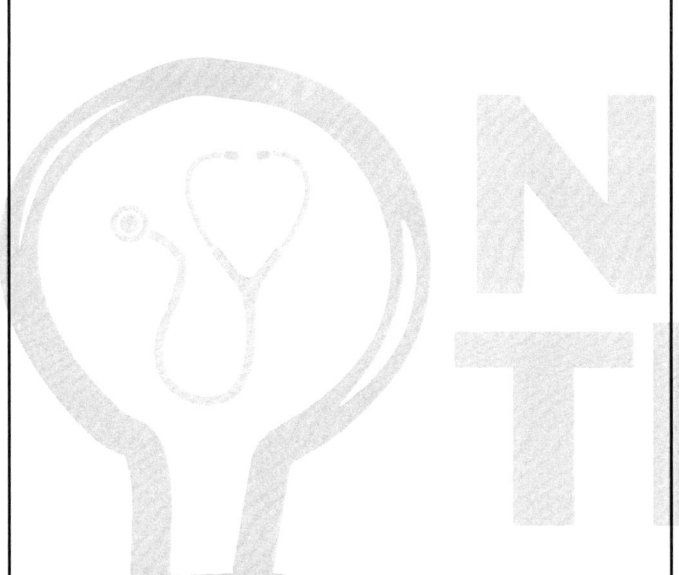

Priority Assessments or Cues	**Priority Labs & Diagnostics**	**Priority Nursing Interventions**
1	1	1
2	2	2
3	3	3

Priority Medications	**Priority Potential & Actual Complications**	**Priority Collaborative Goals**
1	1	1
2	2	2
3	3	3

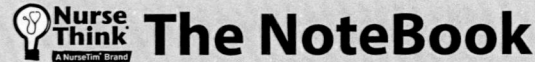
NurseThink® Quick

NEXT GEN LEARNING – NCLEX® TEST PLAN

Safe and Effective Care: Management of Care, Coordinated Care, Safety and Infection Control

Health Promotion and Maintenance

Psychosocial Integrity

Physiological Integrity: Basic Care and Comfort, Pharmacological and Parenteral Therapies, Reduction of Risk Potential, and Physiological Adaptation

QUALITY AND SAFETY COMPETENCIES

Patient-Centered Care

Teamwork and Collaboration

Evidence-Based Practice

Quality Improvement

Safety

Informatics

Peer Review: _____ Faculty Review: _____

Grade Tracker

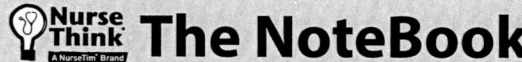
Related Concepts

Related Exemplars/Diseases

Reading/Resources - Clinical Judgment

Class/Lab/Clinical – Clinical Judgment

Priority Assessments or Cues
1
2
3

Priority Labs & Diagnostics
1
2
3

Priority Nursing Interventions
1
2
3

Priority Medications
1
2
3

Priority Potential & Actual Complications
1
2
3

Priority Collaborative Goals
1
2
3

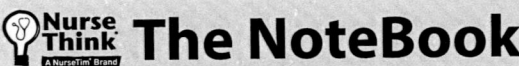
NurseThink® Quick

NEXT GEN LEARNING – NCLEX® TEST PLAN

Safe and Effective Care: Management of Care, Coordinated Care, Safety and Infection Control

Health Promotion and Maintenance

Psychosocial Integrity

Physiological Integrity: Basic Care and Comfort, Pharmacological and Parenteral Therapies, Reduction of Risk Potential, and Physiological Adaptation

QUALITY AND SAFETY COMPETENCIES

Patient-Centered Care

Teamwork and Collaboration

Evidence-Based Practice

Quality Improvement

Safety

Informatics

Peer Review: _____ Faculty Review: _____

Grade Tracker

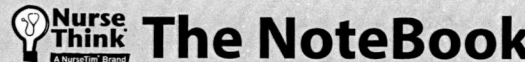
Related Concepts	Related Exemplars/Diseases

Reading/Resources - Clinical Judgment	Class/Lab/Clinical – Clinical Judgment

Priority Assessments or Cues	Priority Labs & Diagnostics	Priority Nursing Interventions
1	1	1
2	2	2
3	3	3

Priority Medications	Priority Potential & Actual Complications	Priority Collaborative Goals
1	1	1
2	2	2
3	3	3

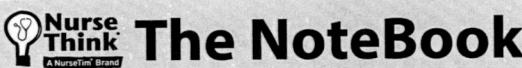
NurseThink® Quick

NEXT GEN LEARNING – NCLEX® TEST PLAN

Safe and Effective Care: Management of Care, Coordinated Care, Safety and Infection Control

Health Promotion and Maintenance

Psychosocial Integrity

Physiological Integrity: Basic Care and Comfort, Pharmacological and Parenteral Therapies, Reduction of Risk Potential, and Physiological Adaptation

QUALITY AND SAFETY COMPETENCIES

Patient-Centered Care

Teamwork and Collaboration

Evidence-Based Practice

Quality Improvement

Safety

Informatics

Peer Review: _____   Faculty Review: _____

Grade Tracker

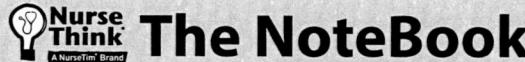
Related Concepts	Related Exemplars/Diseases

Reading/Resources - Clinical Judgment	Class/Lab/Clinical – Clinical Judgment

Priority Assessments or Cues	Priority Labs & Diagnostics	Priority Nursing Interventions
1	1	1
2	2	2
3	3	3

Priority Medications	Priority Potential & Actual Complications	Priority Collaborative Goals
1	1	1
2	2	2
3	3	3

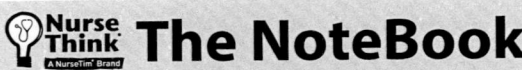
NurseThink® Quick

NEXT GEN LEARNING – NCLEX® TEST PLAN

Safe and Effective Care: Management of Care, Coordinated Care, Safety and Infection Control

Health Promotion and Maintenance

Psychosocial Integrity

Physiological Integrity: Basic Care and Comfort, Pharmacological and Parenteral Therapies, Reduction of Risk Potential, and Physiological Adaptation

QUALITY AND SAFETY COMPETENCIES

Patient-Centered Care

Teamwork and Collaboration

Evidence-Based Practice

Quality Improvement

Safety

Informatics

Peer Review: _____   Faculty Review: _____

Grade Tracker

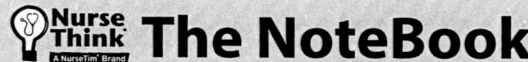

Related Concepts	**Related Exemplars/Diseases**

Reading/Resources - Clinical Judgment	**Class/Lab/Clinical – Clinical Judgment**

Priority Assessments or Cues	**Priority Labs & Diagnostics**	**Priority Nursing Interventions**
1	1	1
2	2	2
3	3	3

Priority Medications	**Priority Potential & Actual Complications**	**Priority Collaborative Goals**
1	1	1
2	2	2
3	3	3

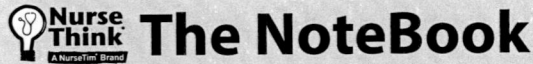
NurseThink® Quick

NEXT GEN LEARNING – NCLEX® TEST PLAN

Safe and Effective Care: Management of Care, Coordinated Care, Safety and Infection Control

Health Promotion and Maintenance

Psychosocial Integrity

Physiological Integrity: Basic Care and Comfort, Pharmacological and Parenteral Therapies, Reduction of Risk Potential, and Physiological Adaptation

QUALITY AND SAFETY COMPETENCIES

Patient-Centered Care

Teamwork and Collaboration

Evidence-Based Practice

Quality Improvement

Safety

Informatics

Peer Review: _____   Faculty Review: _____

Grade Tracker

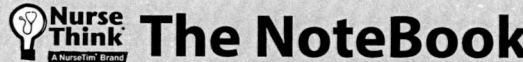

Related Concepts	**Related Exemplars/Diseases**

Reading/Resources - Clinical Judgment	**Class/Lab/Clinical – Clinical Judgment**
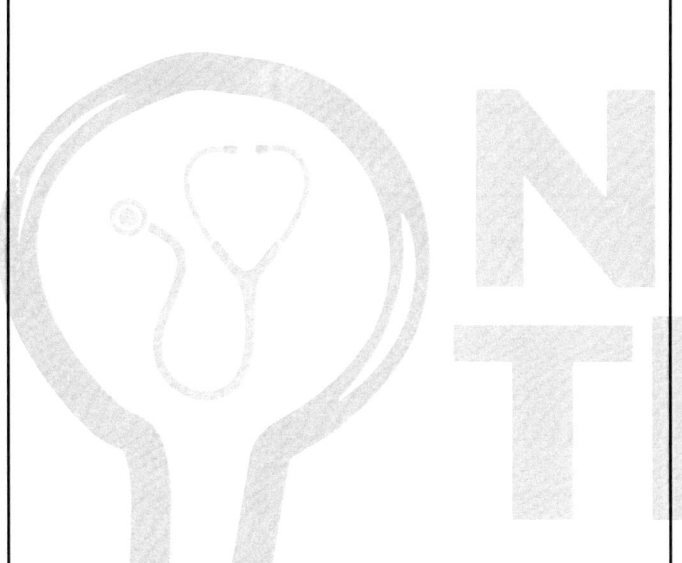	

Priority Assessments or Cues	**Priority Labs & Diagnostics**	**Priority Nursing Interventions**
1	1	1
2	2	2
3	3	3

Priority Medications	**Priority Potential & Actual Complications**	**Priority Collaborative Goals**
1	1	1
2	2	2
3	3	3

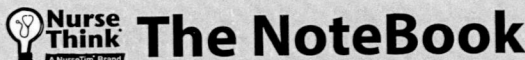
NurseThink® Quick

Cardiomyopathy: Categories
Hard
Hypertrophic
Arrhythmogenic right ventricular
Restrictive
Dilated

NEXT GEN LEARNING – NCLEX® TEST PLAN

Safe and Effective Care: Management of Care, Coordinated Care, Safety and Infection Control

Health Promotion and Maintenance

Psychosocial Integrity

Physiological Integrity: Basic Care and Comfort, Pharmacological and Parenteral Therapies, Reduction of Risk Potential, and Physiological Adaptation

QUALITY AND SAFETY COMPETENCIES

Patient-Centered Care

Teamwork and Collaboration

Evidence-Based Practice

Quality Improvement

Safety

Informatics

Peer Review: _____ Faculty Review: _____

Grade Tracker

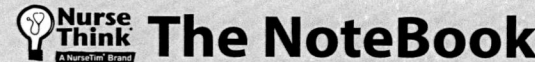

Related Concepts	**Related Exemplars/Diseases**

Reading/Resources - Clinical Judgment	**Class/Lab/Clinical – Clinical Judgment**

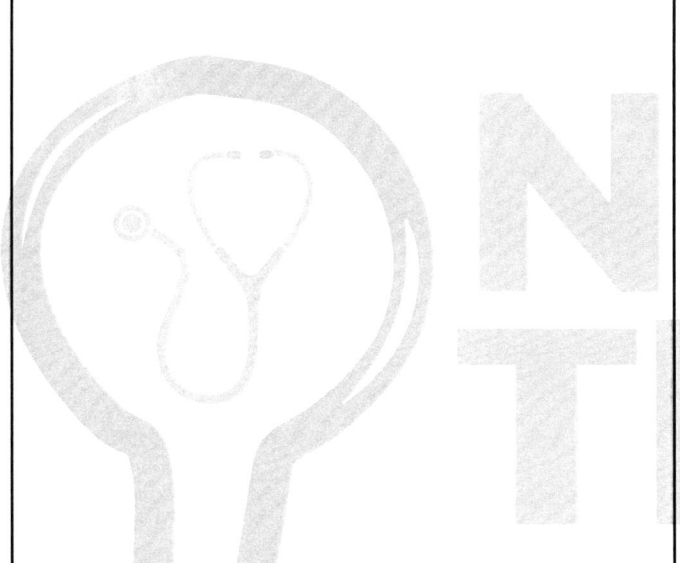

Priority Assessments or Cues	**Priority Labs & Diagnostics**	**Priority Nursing Interventions**
1	1	1
2	2	2
3	3	3

Priority Medications	**Priority Potential & Actual Complications**	**Priority Collaborative Goals**
1	1	1
2	2	2
3	3	3

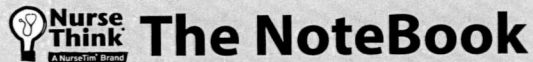
NurseThink® Quick

Digoxin Toxicity	Congestive Heart Failure: Treatment	CHF: Causes of Exacerbation
VANBAD	**Unload Fast**	**Failure**
Vomiting	**U**pright sitting	**F**orgot medication
Anorexia	**N**itroglycerine	**A**rrhythmia/Anemia
Nausea	**L**asix	**I**schemia/Infarction/Infection
Blurred vision	**O**xygen	**L**ifestyle: taken too much salt
Arrhythmias	**A**minophylline	**U**p regulation of cardiac output: pregnancy, hyperthyroidism
Diarrhea	**D**igoxin	**R**enal failure
	Fluids decrease	**E**mbolism: pulmonary
	Afterload decrease	
	Sodium decrease	
	Tests: digoxin Level, ABG, K+, BNP	

NEXT GEN LEARNING – NCLEX® TEST PLAN

Safe and Effective Care: Management of Care, Coordinated Care, Safety and Infection Control

Health Promotion and Maintenance

Psychosocial Integrity

Physiological Integrity: Basic Care and Comfort, Pharmacological and Parenteral Therapies, Reduction of Risk Potential, and Physiological Adaptation

QUALITY AND SAFETY COMPETENCIES

Patient-Centered Care

Teamwork and Collaboration

Evidence-Based Practice

Quality Improvement

Safety

Informatics

Peer Review: _____   Faculty Review: _____

Grade Tracker

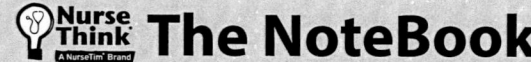

Related Concepts

Related Exemplars/Diseases

Reading/Resources - Clinical Judgment

Class/Lab/Clinical – Clinical Judgment

Priority Assessments or Cues

1

2

3

Priority Labs & Diagnostics

1

2

3

Priority Nursing Interventions

1

2

3

Priority Medications

1

2

3

**Priority Potential &
Actual Complications**

1

2

3

Priority Collaborative Goals

1

2

3

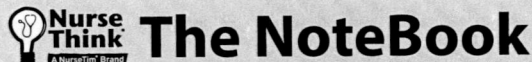
NurseThink® Quick

Hypertension Complications
4 C's
Coronary artery disease
Congestive heart failure
Chronic renal failure
Cardiovascular accident

Hypertension Treatment
ABCD
ACE inhibitors/AngII antagonists
Beta blockers
Calcium antagonists
Diuretics/ Vasodilators

Hypertension Interventions
I-Tired
Intake and output
Transient ischemic attack (monitor)
Impaired perfusion monitoring
Respiration, pulse
Electrolytes
Daily weight

Hypertension: Secondary HTN Causes:
Chaps
Cushing's syndrome
Hyperaldosteronism
Aorta coarctation
Pheochromocytoma
Stenosis of renal arteries

NEXT GEN LEARNING – NCLEX® TEST PLAN

Safe and Effective Care: Management of Care, Coordinated Care, Safety and Infection Control

Health Promotion and Maintenance

Psychosocial Integrity

Physiological Integrity: Basic Care and Comfort, Pharmacological and Parenteral Therapies, Reduction of Risk Potential, and Physiological Adaptation

QUALITY AND SAFETY COMPETENCIES

Patient-Centered Care

Teamwork and Collaboration

Evidence-Based Practice

Quality Improvement

Safety

Informatics

Peer Review: _____   Faculty Review: _____

Grade Tracker

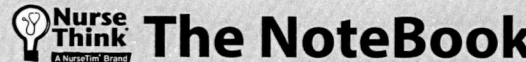

Related Concepts	Related Exemplars/Diseases

Reading/Resources - Clinical Judgment	Class/Lab/Clinical – Clinical Judgment

Priority Assessments or Cues	Priority Labs & Diagnostics	Priority Nursing Interventions
1	1	1
2	2	2
3	3	3

Priority Medications	Priority Potential & Actual Complications	Priority Collaborative Goals
1	1	1
2	2	2
3	3	3

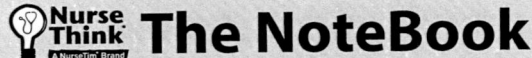
NurseThink® Quick

Myocardial Infarction: Signs and Symptoms
Pulse
Persistent chest pains
Upset stomach
Lightheadedness
Shortness of breath
Excessive sweating

Myocardial Infarction: Treatment
Monah
Morphine sulfate
Oxygen
Nitroglycerin
ASA
Heparin

MI: Complications
Leap on the Map
LVF
Embolism
Aneurysm
Progressive infarct
Myocardial rupture
Arrhythmias
Pericarditis

Myocardial Infarction: Management
Boomar
Bedrest
Oxygen
Opiate
Monitor
Anticoagulant
Reduce clot size

NEXT GEN LEARNING – NCLEX® TEST PLAN

Safe and Effective Care: Management of Care, Coordinated Care, Safety and Infection Control

Health Promotion and Maintenance

Psychosocial Integrity

Physiological Integrity: Basic Care and Comfort, Pharmacological and Parenteral Therapies, Reduction of Risk Potential, and Physiological Adaptation

---

QUALITY AND SAFETY COMPETENCIES

Patient-Centered Care

Teamwork and Collaboration

Evidence-Based Practice

Quality Improvement

Safety

Informatics

Peer Review: _____   Faculty Review: _____

Grade Tracker

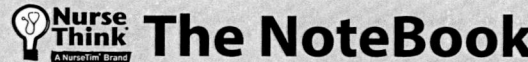

Related Concepts

Related Exemplars/Diseases

Reading/Resources - Clinical Judgment

Class/Lab/Clinical – Clinical Judgment

Priority Assessments or Cues

1

2

3

Priority Labs & Diagnostics

1

2

3

Priority Nursing Interventions

1

2

3

Priority Medications

1

2

3

Priority Potential & Actual Complications

1

2

3

Priority Collaborative Goals

1

2

3

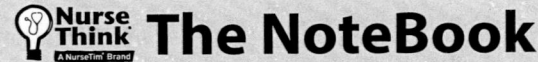
NurseThink® Quick

Aortic Stenosis Characteristics
SAD
Syncope
Angina
Dyspnea

Mitral Stenosis (MS) vs. Regurgitation (MR)
MS is a female predominant
MR is male predominant

Murmur Attributes
IL PQRST
Intensity
Location
Pitch
Quality
Radiation
Shape
Timing

Mitral Stenosis: Complications
ABCED x 2
Arrhythmias/Aneurysm
Bradycardia/Low BP
Cardiac Failure/Cardiac tamponade
Dresslers/Death
Embolism

NEXT GEN LEARNING – NCLEX® TEST PLAN

Safe and Effective Care: Management of Care, Coordinated Care, Safety and Infection Control

Health Promotion and Maintenance

Psychosocial Integrity

Physiological Integrity: Basic Care and Comfort, Pharmacological and Parenteral Therapies, Reduction of Risk Potential, and Physiological Adaptation

QUALITY AND SAFETY COMPETENCIES

Patient-Centered Care

Teamwork and Collaboration

Evidence-Based Practice

Quality Improvement

Safety

Informatics

Peer Review: _____   Faculty Review: _____

Grade Tracker

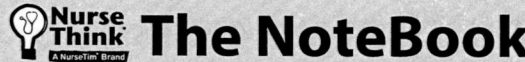

Related Concepts	Related Exemplars/Diseases

Reading/Resources - Clinical Judgment	Class/Lab/Clinical – Clinical Judgment

Priority Assessments or Cues	Priority Labs & Diagnostics	Priority Nursing Interventions
1	1	1
2	2	2
3	3	3

Priority Medications	Priority Potential & Actual Complications	Priority Collaborative Goals
1	1	1
2	2	2
3	3	3

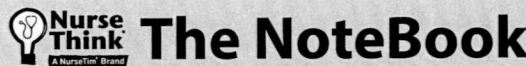
NurseThink® Quick

NEXT GEN LEARNING – NCLEX® TEST PLAN

Safe and Effective Care: Management of Care, Coordinated Care, Safety and Infection Control

Health Promotion and Maintenance

Psychosocial Integrity

Physiological Integrity: Basic Care and Comfort, Pharmacological and Parenteral Therapies, Reduction of Risk Potential, and Physiological Adaptation

QUALITY AND SAFETY COMPETENCIES

Patient-Centered Care

Teamwork and Collaboration

Evidence-Based Practice

Quality Improvement

Safety

Informatics

Peer Review: _____   Faculty Review: _____

Grade Tracker

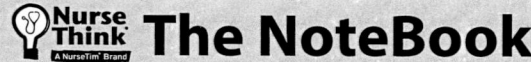

Related Concepts	Related Exemplars/Diseases

Reading/Resources - Clinical Judgment	Class/Lab/Clinical – Clinical Judgment

Priority Assessments or Cues	Priority Labs & Diagnostics	Priority Nursing Interventions
1	1	1
2	2	2
3	3	3

Priority Medications	Priority Potential & Actual Complications	Priority Collaborative Goals
1	1	1
2	2	2
3	3	3

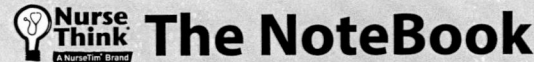
NurseThink® Quick

NEXT GEN LEARNING – NCLEX® TEST PLAN

Safe and Effective Care: Management of Care, Coordinated Care, Safety and Infection Control

Health Promotion and Maintenance

Psychosocial Integrity

Physiological Integrity: Basic Care and Comfort, Pharmacological and Parenteral Therapies, Reduction of Risk Potential, and Physiological Adaptation

QUALITY AND SAFETY COMPETENCIES

Patient-Centered Care

Teamwork and Collaboration

Evidence-Based Practice

Quality Improvement

Safety

Informatics

Peer Review: _____ Faculty Review: _____

Grade Tracker

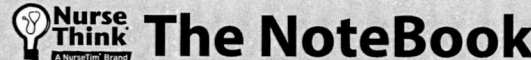
Related Concepts	Related Exemplars/Diseases

Reading/Resources - Clinical Judgment	Class/Lab/Clinical – Clinical Judgment

Priority Assessments or Cues
1
2
3

Priority Labs & Diagnostics
1
2
3

Priority Nursing Interventions
1
2
3

Priority Medications
1
2
3

Priority Potential & Actual Complications
1
2
3

Priority Collaborative Goals
1
2
3

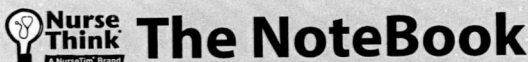
NurseThink® Quick

NEXT GEN LEARNING – NCLEX® TEST PLAN

Safe and Effective Care: Management of Care, Coordinated Care, Safety and Infection Control

Health Promotion and Maintenance

Psychosocial Integrity

Physiological Integrity: Basic Care and Comfort, Pharmacological and Parenteral Therapies, Reduction of Risk Potential, and Physiological Adaptation

QUALITY AND SAFETY COMPETENCIES

Patient-Centered Care

Teamwork and Collaboration

Evidence-Based Practice

Quality Improvement

Safety

Informatics

Peer Review: _____   Faculty Review: _____

Grade Tracker

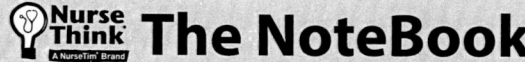
Related Concepts	**Related Exemplars/Diseases**

Reading/Resources - Clinical Judgment	**Class/Lab/Clinical – Clinical Judgment**
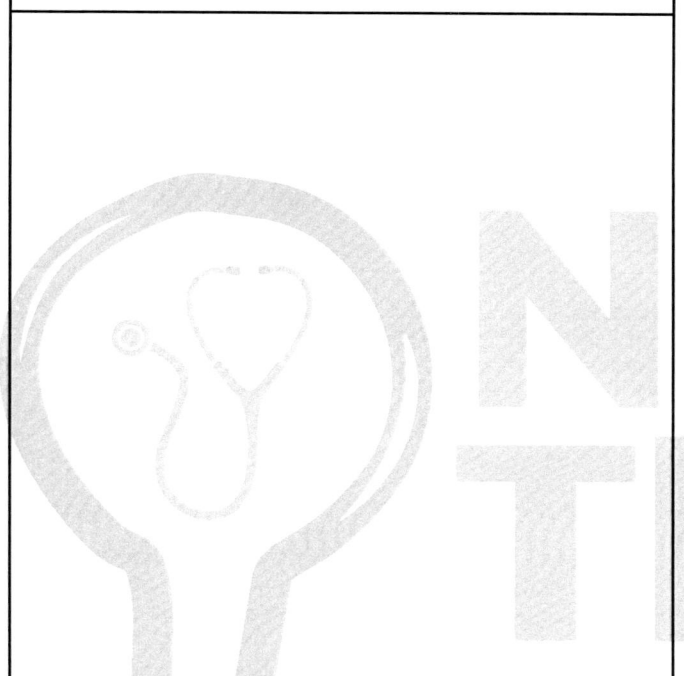	

Priority Assessments or Cues	**Priority Labs & Diagnostics**	**Priority Nursing Interventions**
1	1	1
2	2	2
3	3	3

Priority Medications	**Priority Potential & Actual Complications**	**Priority Collaborative Goals**
1	1	1
2	2	2
3	3	3

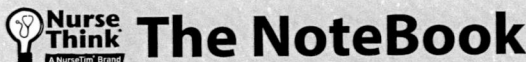

NurseThink® Quick

NEXT GEN LEARNING – NCLEX® TEST PLAN

Safe and Effective Care: Management of Care, Coordinated Care, Safety and Infection Control

Health Promotion and Maintenance

Psychosocial Integrity

Physiological Integrity: Basic Care and Comfort, Pharmacological and Parenteral Therapies, Reduction of Risk Potential, and Physiological Adaptation

QUALITY AND SAFETY COMPETENCIES

Patient-Centered Care

Teamwork and Collaboration

Evidence-Based Practice

Quality Improvement

Safety

Informatics

Peer Review: _____ Faculty Review: _____

Grade Tracker

Related Concepts

Related Exemplars/Diseases

Reading/Resources - Clinical Judgment

Class/Lab/Clinical – Clinical Judgment

Priority Assessments or Cues

1

2

3

Priority Labs & Diagnostics

1

2

3

Priority Nursing Interventions

1

2

3

Priority Medications

1

2

3

Priority Potential & Actual Complications

1

2

3

Priority Collaborative Goals

1

2

3

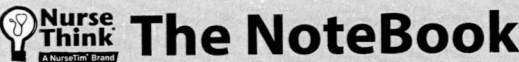
NurseThink® Quick

NEXT GEN LEARNING – NCLEX® TEST PLAN

Safe and Effective Care: Management of Care, Coordinated Care, Safety and Infection Control

Health Promotion and Maintenance

Psychosocial Integrity

Physiological Integrity: Basic Care and Comfort, Pharmacological and Parenteral Therapies, Reduction of Risk Potential, and Physiological Adaptation

QUALITY AND SAFETY COMPETENCIES

Patient-Centered Care

Teamwork and Collaboration

Evidence-Based Practice

Quality Improvement

Safety

Informatics

Peer Review: _____   Faculty Review: _____

Grade Tracker

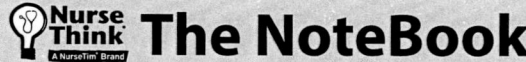
Related Concepts

Related Exemplars/Diseases

Reading/Resources - Clinical Judgment

Class/Lab/Clinical – Clinical Judgment

Priority Assessments or Cues

1
2
3

Priority Labs & Diagnostics

1
2
3

Priority Nursing Interventions

1
2
3

Priority Medications

1
2
3

Priority Potential & Actual Complications

1
2
3

Priority Collaborative Goals

1
2
3

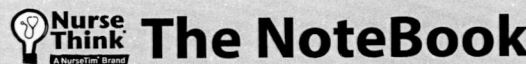
NurseThink® Quick

NEXT GEN LEARNING – NCLEX® TEST PLAN

Safe and Effective Care: Management of Care, Coordinated Care, Safety and Infection Control

Health Promotion and Maintenance

Psychosocial Integrity

Physiological Integrity: Basic Care and Comfort, Pharmacological and Parenteral Therapies, Reduction of Risk Potential, and Physiological Adaptation

QUALITY AND SAFETY COMPETENCIES

Patient-Centered Care

Teamwork and Collaboration

Evidence-Based Practice

Quality Improvement

Safety

Informatics

Peer Review: _____   Faculty Review: _____

Grade Tracker

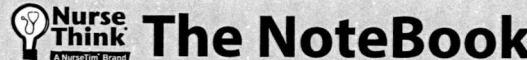
Related Concepts	Related Exemplars/Diseases

Reading/Resources - Clinical Judgment	Class/Lab/Clinical – Clinical Judgment

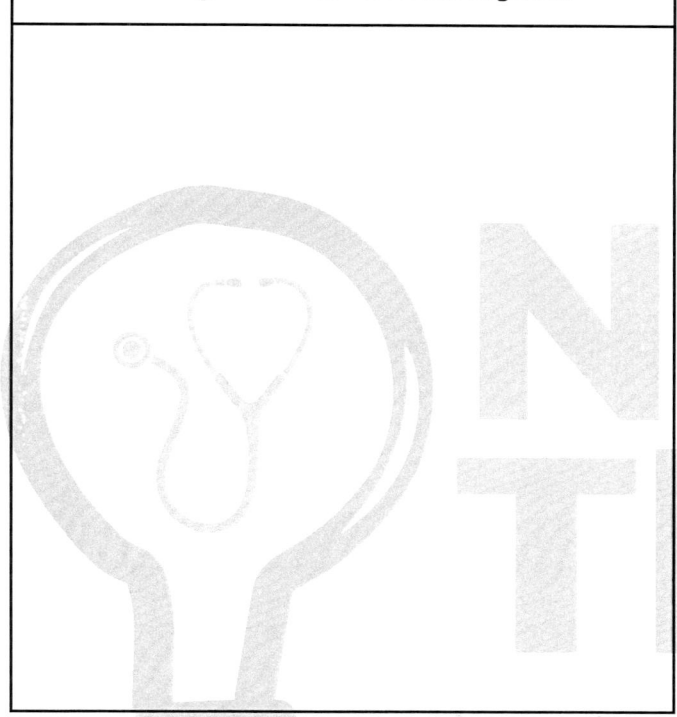

Priority Assessments or Cues
1
2
3

Priority Labs & Diagnostics
1
2
3

Priority Nursing Interventions
1
2
3

Priority Medications
1
2
3

Priority Potential & Actual Complications
1
2
3

Priority Collaborative Goals
1
2
3

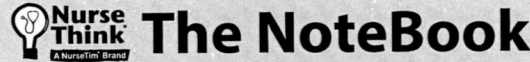
NurseThink® Quick

<table>
<tr><td></td><td></td><td></td></tr>
</table>

NEXT GEN LEARNING – NCLEX® TEST PLAN

Safe and Effective Care: Management of Care, Coordinated Care, Safety and Infection Control

Health Promotion and Maintenance

Psychosocial Integrity

Physiological Integrity: Basic Care and Comfort, Pharmacological and Parenteral Therapies, Reduction of Risk Potential, and Physiological Adaptation

QUALITY AND SAFETY COMPETENCIES

Patient-Centered Care

Teamwork and Collaboration

Evidence-Based Practice

Quality Improvement

Safety

Informatics

Peer Review: _____   Faculty Review: _____

Grade Tracker

<table>
<tr><td></td><td></td><td></td><td></td><td></td><td></td><td></td><td></td><td></td><td></td><td></td><td></td><td></td><td></td><td></td><td></td></tr>
</table>

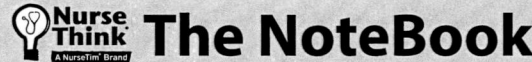

Related Concepts	Related Exemplars/Diseases

Reading/Resources - Clinical Judgment	Class/Lab/Clinical – Clinical Judgment
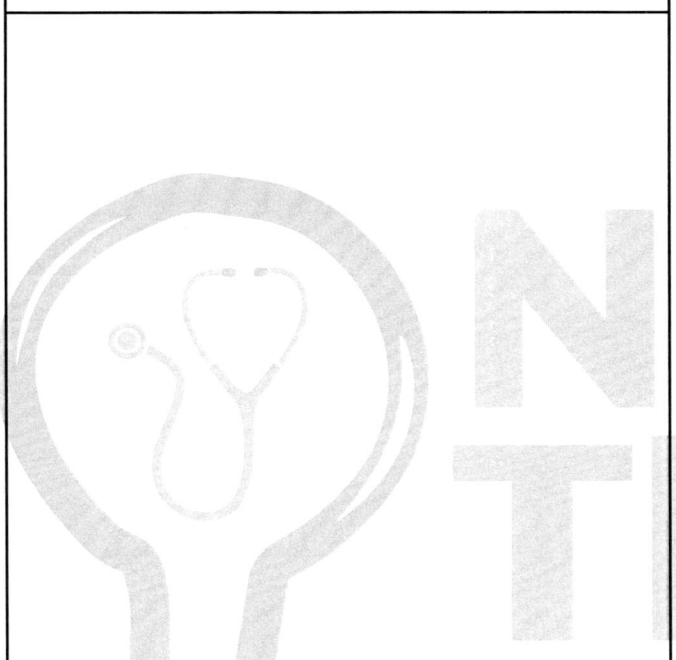	

Priority Assessments or Cues	Priority Labs & Diagnostics	Priority Nursing Interventions
1	1	1
2	2	2
3	3	3

Priority Medications	Priority Potential & Actual Complications	Priority Collaborative Goals
1	1	1
2	2	2
3	3	3

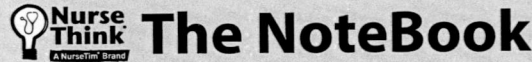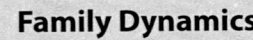
NurseThink® Quick

NEXT GEN LEARNING – NCLEX® TEST PLAN

Safe and Effective Care: Management of Care, Coordinated Care, Safety and Infection Control

Health Promotion and Maintenance

Psychosocial Integrity

Physiological Integrity: Basic Care and Comfort, Pharmacological and Parenteral Therapies, Reduction of Risk Potential, and Physiological Adaptation

QUALITY AND SAFETY COMPETENCIES

Patient-Centered Care

Teamwork and Collaboration

Evidence-Based Practice

Quality Improvement

Safety

Informatics

Peer Review: _____   Faculty Review: _____

Grade Tracker

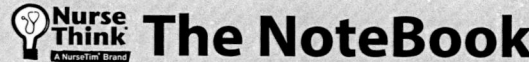
Related Concepts	**Related Exemplars/Diseases**

Reading/Resources - Clinical Judgment	**Class/Lab/Clinical – Clinical Judgment**

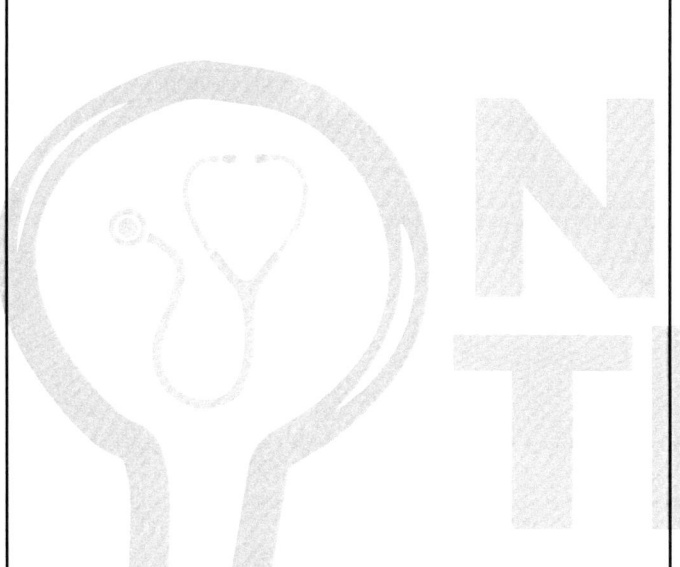

Priority Assessments or Cues	**Priority Labs & Diagnostics**	**Priority Nursing Interventions**
1	1	1
2	2	2
3	3	3

Priority Medications	**Priority Potential & Actual Complications**	**Priority Collaborative Goals**
1	1	1
2	2	2
3	3	3

NurseThink® Quick

NEXT GEN LEARNING – NCLEX® TEST PLAN

Safe and Effective Care: Management of Care, Coordinated Care, Safety and Infection Control

Health Promotion and Maintenance

Psychosocial Integrity

Physiological Integrity: Basic Care and Comfort, Pharmacological and Parenteral Therapies, Reduction of Risk Potential, and Physiological Adaptation

QUALITY AND SAFETY COMPETENCIES

Patient-Centered Care

Teamwork and Collaboration

Evidence-Based Practice

Quality Improvement

Safety

Informatics

Peer Review: _____   Faculty Review: _____

Grade Tracker

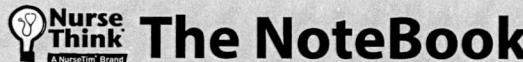

Related Concepts	**Related Exemplars/Diseases**

Reading/Resources - Clinical Judgment	**Class/Lab/Clinical – Clinical Judgment**

Priority Assessments or Cues	**Priority Labs & Diagnostics**	**Priority Nursing Interventions**
1	1	1
2	2	2
3	3	3

Priority Medications	**Priority Potential & Actual Complications**	**Priority Collaborative Goals**
1	1	1
2	2	2
3	3	3

NurseThink® Quick

NEXT GEN LEARNING – NCLEX® TEST PLAN

Safe and Effective Care: Management of Care, Coordinated Care, Safety and Infection Control

Health Promotion and Maintenance

Psychosocial Integrity

Physiological Integrity: Basic Care and Comfort, Pharmacological and Parenteral Therapies, Reduction of Risk Potential, and Physiological Adaptation

QUALITY AND SAFETY COMPETENCIES

Patient-Centered Care

Teamwork and Collaboration

Evidence-Based Practice

Quality Improvement

Safety

Informatics

Peer Review: _____ Faculty Review: _____

Grade Tracker

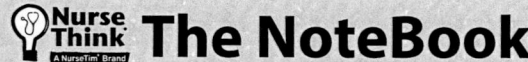

Related Concepts	Related Exemplars/Diseases

Reading/Resources - Clinical Judgment	Class/Lab/Clinical – Clinical Judgment

Priority Assessments or Cues	Priority Labs & Diagnostics	Priority Nursing Interventions
1	1	1
2	2	2
3	3	3

Priority Medications	Priority Potential & Actual Complications	Priority Collaborative Goals
1	1	1
2	2	2
3	3	3

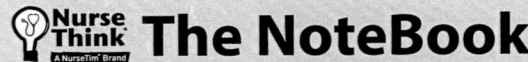

NurseThink® Quick

┌─────────────────┬─────────────────┬─────────────────┐
│   │   │   │
│   │   │   │
│   │   │   │
│   │   │   │
│   │   │   │
│   │   │   │
└─────────────────┴─────────────────┴─────────────────┘

NEXT GEN LEARNING – NCLEX® TEST PLAN

Safe and Effective Care: Management of Care, Coordinated Care, Safety and Infection Control

Health Promotion and Maintenance

Psychosocial Integrity

Physiological Integrity: Basic Care and Comfort, Pharmacological and Parenteral Therapies, Reduction of Risk Potential, and Physiological Adaptation

QUALITY AND SAFETY COMPETENCIES

Patient-Centered Care

Teamwork and Collaboration

Evidence-Based Practice

Quality Improvement

Safety

Informatics

Peer Review: _____   Faculty Review: _____

Grade Tracker

┌──┬──┬──┬──┬──┬──┬──┬──┬──┬──┬──┬──┬──┬──┬──┬──┬──┬──┬──┐
│ │ │ │ │ │ │ │ │ │ │ │ │ │ │ │ │ │ │ │
└──┴──┴──┴──┴──┴──┴──┴──┴──┴──┴──┴──┴──┴──┴──┴──┴──┴──┴──┘

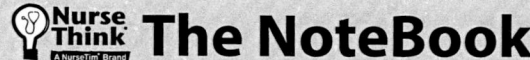
Related Concepts	**Related Exemplars/Diseases**

Reading/Resources - Clinical Judgment	**Class/Lab/Clinical – Clinical Judgment**

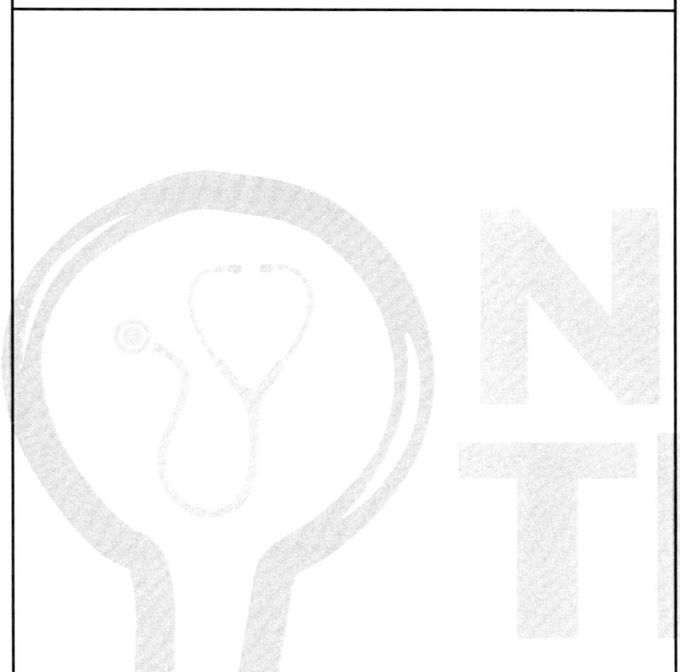

Priority Assessments or Cues	**Priority Labs & Diagnostics**	**Priority Nursing Interventions**
1	1	1
2	2	2
3	3	3

Priority Medications	**Priority Potential & Actual Complications**	**Priority Collaborative Goals**
1	1	1
2	2	2
3	3	3

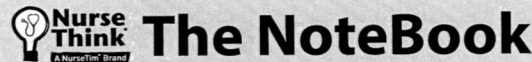
NurseThink® Quick

NEXT GEN LEARNING – NCLEX® TEST PLAN

Safe and Effective Care: Management of Care, Coordinated Care, Safety and Infection Control

Health Promotion and Maintenance

Psychosocial Integrity

Physiological Integrity: Basic Care and Comfort, Pharmacological and Parenteral Therapies, Reduction of Risk Potential, and Physiological Adaptation

QUALITY AND SAFETY COMPETENCIES

Patient-Centered Care

Teamwork and Collaboration

Evidence-Based Practice

Quality Improvement

Safety

Informatics

Peer Review: _____   Faculty Review: _____

Grade Tracker

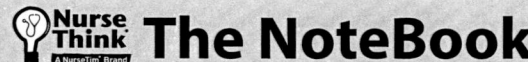
Related Concepts	**Related Exemplars/Diseases**

Reading/Resources - Clinical Judgment	**Class/Lab/Clinical – Clinical Judgment**

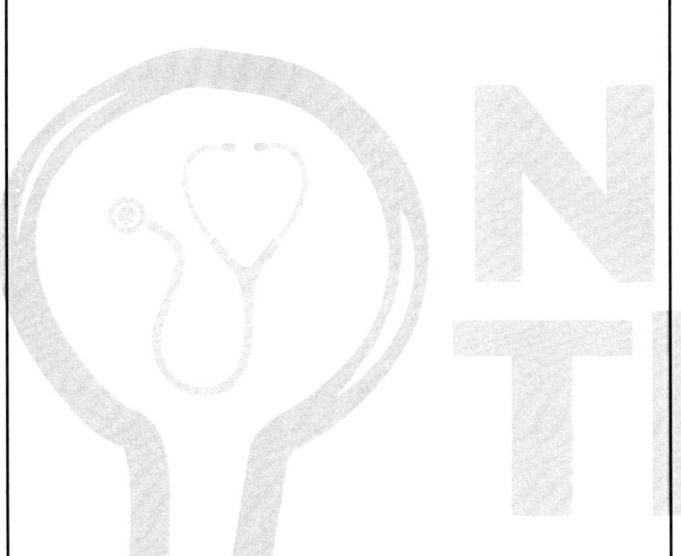

Priority Assessments or Cues	**Priority Labs & Diagnostics**	**Priority Nursing Interventions**
1	1	1
2	2	2
3	3	3

Priority Medications	**Priority Potential & Actual Complications**	**Priority Collaborative Goals**
1	1	1
2	2	2
3	3	3

⚬NurseThink The NoteBook

NurseThink® Quick

NEXT GEN LEARNING – NCLEX® TEST PLAN

Safe and Effective Care: Management of Care, Coordinated Care, Safety and Infection Control

Health Promotion and Maintenance

Psychosocial Integrity

Physiological Integrity: Basic Care and Comfort, Pharmacological and Parenteral Therapies, Reduction of Risk Potential, and Physiological Adaptation

QUALITY AND SAFETY COMPETENCIES

Patient-Centered Care

Teamwork and Collaboration

Evidence-Based Practice

Quality Improvement

Safety

Informatics

Peer Review: _____   Faculty Review: _____

Grade Tracker

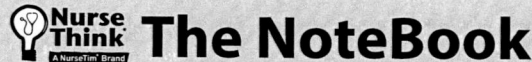
Related Concepts	**Related Exemplars/Diseases**

Reading/Resources - Clinical Judgment	**Class/Lab/Clinical – Clinical Judgment**

Priority Assessments or Cues	**Priority Labs & Diagnostics**	**Priority Nursing Interventions**
1	1	1
2	2	2
3	3	3

Priority Medications	**Priority Potential & Actual Complications**	**Priority Collaborative Goals**
1	1	1
2	2	2
3	3	3

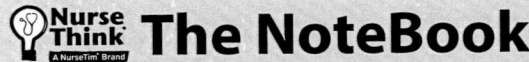
NurseThink® Quick

NEXT GEN LEARNING – NCLEX® TEST PLAN

Safe and Effective Care: Management of Care, Coordinated Care, Safety and Infection Control

Health Promotion and Maintenance

Psychosocial Integrity

Physiological Integrity: Basic Care and Comfort, Pharmacological and Parenteral Therapies, Reduction of Risk Potential, and Physiological Adaptation

QUALITY AND SAFETY COMPETENCIES

Patient-Centered Care

Teamwork and Collaboration

Evidence-Based Practice

Quality Improvement

Safety

Informatics

Peer Review: _____ Faculty Review: _____

Grade Tracker

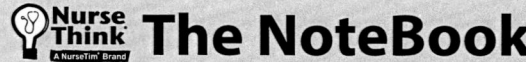
Related Concepts	Related Exemplars/Diseases

Reading/Resources - Clinical Judgment	Class/Lab/Clinical – Clinical Judgment

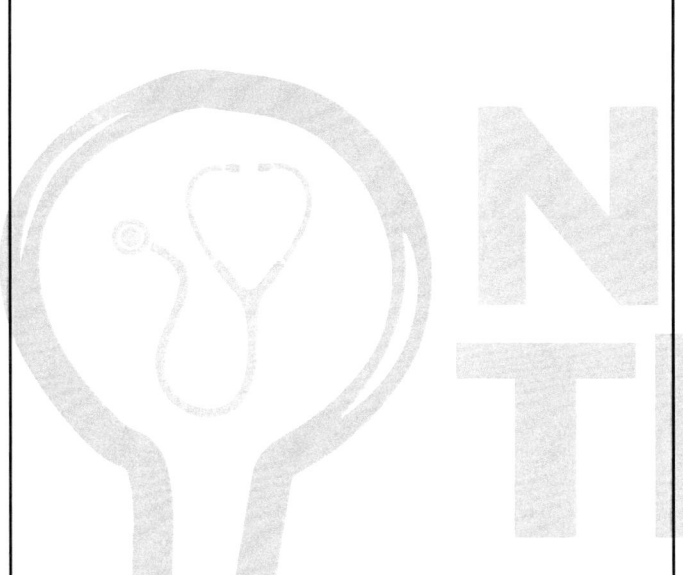

Priority Assessments or Cues	Priority Labs & Diagnostics	Priority Nursing Interventions
1	1	1
2	2	2
3	3	3

Priority Medications	Priority Potential & Actual Complications	Priority Collaborative Goals
1	1	1
2	2	2
3	3	3

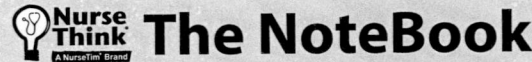
NurseThink® Quick

NEXT GEN LEARNING – NCLEX® TEST PLAN

Safe and Effective Care: Management of Care, Coordinated Care, Safety and Infection Control

Health Promotion and Maintenance

Psychosocial Integrity

Physiological Integrity: Basic Care and Comfort, Pharmacological and Parenteral Therapies, Reduction of Risk Potential, and Physiological Adaptation

QUALITY AND SAFETY COMPETENCIES

Patient-Centered Care

Teamwork and Collaboration

Evidence-Based Practice

Quality Improvement

Safety

Informatics

Peer Review: _____   Faculty Review: _____

Grade Tracker

Related Concepts

Related Exemplars/Diseases

Reading/Resources - Clinical Judgment

Class/Lab/Clinical – Clinical Judgment

Priority Assessments or Cues

1

2

3

Priority Labs & Diagnostics

1

2

3

Priority Nursing Interventions

1

2

3

Priority Medications

1

2

3

Priority Potential & Actual Complications

1

2

3

Priority Collaborative Goals

1

2

3

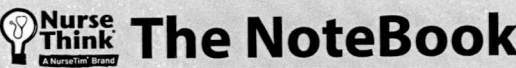
NurseThink® Quick

NEXT GEN LEARNING – NCLEX® TEST PLAN

Safe and Effective Care: Management of Care, Coordinated Care, Safety and Infection Control

Health Promotion and Maintenance

Psychosocial Integrity

Physiological Integrity: Basic Care and Comfort, Pharmacological and Parenteral Therapies, Reduction of Risk Potential, and Physiological Adaptation

QUALITY AND SAFETY COMPETENCIES

Patient-Centered Care

Teamwork and Collaboration

Evidence-Based Practice

Quality Improvement

Safety

Informatics

Peer Review: _____   Faculty Review: _____

Grade Tracker

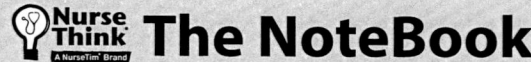

Related Concepts

Related Exemplars/Diseases

Reading/Resources - Clinical Judgment

Class/Lab/Clinical – Clinical Judgment

Priority Assessments or Cues

1
2
3

Priority Labs & Diagnostics

1
2
3

Priority Nursing Interventions

1
2
3

Priority Medications

1
2
3

Priority Potential & Actual Complications

1
2
3

Priority Collaborative Goals

1
2
3

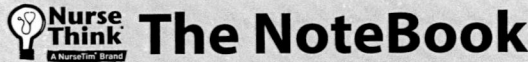
NurseThink® Quick

Altered Mental State: Causes	Confusion: Causes	
AEIOU Tips **A**lcohol/Drugs **E**ndocrine **I**nsulin **U**remia **O**verdose **T**oxins/Trauma/Tumor **I**nfections **P**sychosis/Porphyria **S**troke/Seizure/Shock	**Dim Face** **D**rugs Dehydration **I**nfection **M**etabolic/MI **F**racture/Failure **A**lcohol/Anemia **C**VA **E**lectrolyte disturbances	

NEXT GEN LEARNING – NCLEX® TEST PLAN

Safe and Effective Care: Management of Care, Coordinated Care, Safety and Infection Control

Health Promotion and Maintenance

Psychosocial Integrity

Physiological Integrity: Basic Care and Comfort, Pharmacological and Parenteral Therapies, Reduction of Risk Potential, and Physiological Adaptation

QUALITY AND SAFETY COMPETENCIES

Patient-Centered Care

Teamwork and Collaboration

Evidence-Based Practice

Quality Improvement

Safety

Informatics

Peer Review: _____　　　Faculty Review: _____

Grade Tracker

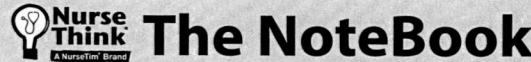
Related Concepts	Related Exemplars/Diseases

Reading/Resources - Clinical Judgment	Class/Lab/Clinical – Clinical Judgment

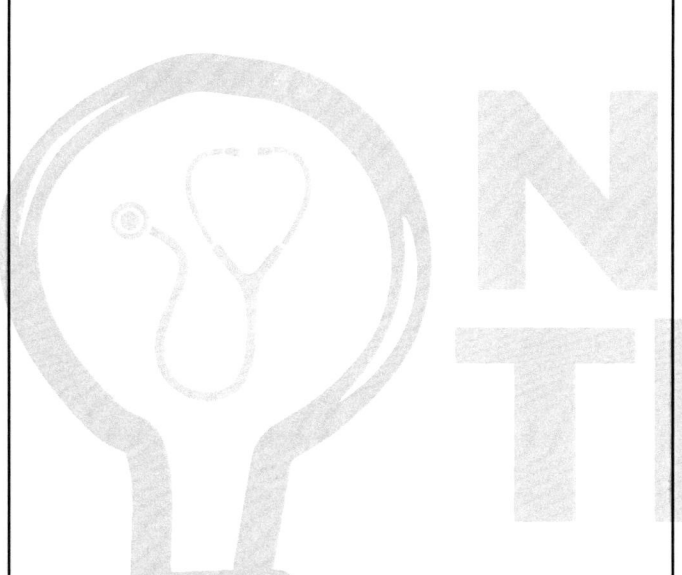

Priority Assessments or Cues	Priority Labs & Diagnostics	Priority Nursing Interventions
1	1	1
2	2	2
3	3	3

Priority Medications	Priority Potential & Actual Complications	Priority Collaborative Goals
1	1	1
2	2	2
3	3	3

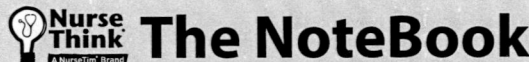

NurseThink® Quick

Dementia: Causes ***Dementia*** **D**rugs and alcohol (including over-the-counter drugs) **E**yes and ears (disorientation due to visual/auditory distortion) **M**edical disorders (diabetes, hypothyroidism) **E**motional and psychological disturbances (mood or paranoid disorders) **N**eurological disorders (multiinfarct dementia) **T**umors and trauma **I**nfections (urinary tract or upper respiratory tract) **A**rteriosclerosis (leading to heart failure, insufficient blood supply to heart and brain, and confusion)	**Alzheimer's Disease: Progressive Phases** ***ABCD*** **A**mnesic phase (forgetting) **B**ehavioral problems (antisocial, wandering) **C**ortical phase (incontinence, falls) **D**ecerebrate phase (return to primitive reflexes)	

NEXT GEN LEARNING – NCLEX® TEST PLAN

Safe and Effective Care: Management of Care, Coordinated Care, Safety and Infection Control

Health Promotion and Maintenance

Psychosocial Integrity

Physiological Integrity: Basic Care and Comfort, Pharmacological and Parenteral Therapies, Reduction of Risk Potential, and Physiological Adaptation

QUALITY AND SAFETY COMPETENCIES

Patient-Centered Care

Teamwork and Collaboration

Evidence-Based Practice

Quality Improvement

Safety

Informatics

Peer Review: _____   Faculty Review: _____

Grade Tracker

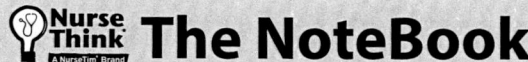
Related Concepts

Related Exemplars/Diseases

Reading/Resources - Clinical Judgment

Class/Lab/Clinical – Clinical Judgment

Priority Assessments or Cues

1

2

3

Priority Labs & Diagnostics

1

2

3

Priority Nursing Interventions

1

2

3

Priority Medications

1

2

3

Priority Potential & Actual Complications

1

2

3

Priority Collaborative Goals

1

2

3

NurseThink® Quick

NEXT GEN LEARNING – NCLEX® TEST PLAN

Safe and Effective Care: Management of Care, Coordinated Care, Safety and Infection Control

Health Promotion and Maintenance

Psychosocial Integrity

Physiological Integrity: Basic Care and Comfort, Pharmacological and Parenteral Therapies, Reduction of Risk Potential, and Physiological Adaptation

QUALITY AND SAFETY COMPETENCIES

Patient-Centered Care

Teamwork and Collaboration

Evidence-Based Practice

Quality Improvement

Safety

Informatics

Peer Review: _____   Faculty Review: _____

Grade Tracker

NurseThink The NoteBook

Related Concepts

Related Exemplars/Diseases

Reading/Resources - Clinical Judgment

Class/Lab/Clinical – Clinical Judgment

Priority Assessments or Cues

1

2

3

Priority Labs & Diagnostics

1

2

3

Priority Nursing Interventions

1

2

3

Priority Medications

1

2

3

Priority Potential & Actual Complications

1

2

3

Priority Collaborative Goals

1

2

3

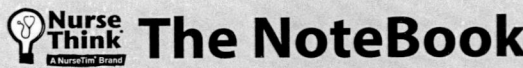
NurseThink® Quick

NEXT GEN LEARNING – NCLEX® TEST PLAN

Safe and Effective Care: Management of Care, Coordinated Care, Safety and Infection Control

Health Promotion and Maintenance

Psychosocial Integrity

Physiological Integrity: Basic Care and Comfort, Pharmacological and Parenteral Therapies, Reduction of Risk Potential, and Physiological Adaptation

QUALITY AND SAFETY COMPETENCIES

Patient-Centered Care

Teamwork and Collaboration

Evidence-Based Practice

Quality Improvement

Safety

Informatics

Peer Review: _____   Faculty Review: _____

Grade Tracker

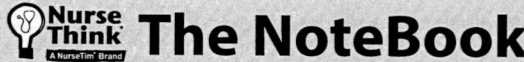

Related Concepts	Related Exemplars/Diseases

Reading/Resources - Clinical Judgment	Class/Lab/Clinical – Clinical Judgment

Priority Assessments or Cues	Priority Labs & Diagnostics	Priority Nursing Interventions
1	1	1
2	2	2
3	3	3

Priority Medications	Priority Potential & Actual Complications	Priority Collaborative Goals
1	1	1
2	2	2
3	3	3

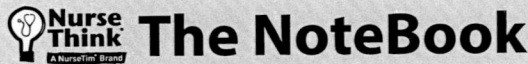
NurseThink® Quick

NEXT GEN LEARNING – NCLEX® TEST PLAN

Safe and Effective Care: Management of Care, Coordinated Care, Safety and Infection Control

Health Promotion and Maintenance

Psychosocial Integrity

Physiological Integrity: Basic Care and Comfort, Pharmacological and Parenteral Therapies, Reduction of Risk Potential, and Physiological Adaptation

QUALITY AND SAFETY COMPETENCIES

Patient-Centered Care

Teamwork and Collaboration

Evidence-Based Practice

Quality Improvement

Safety

Informatics

Peer Review: _____   Faculty Review: _____

Grade Tracker

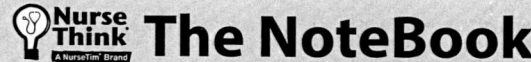

Related Concepts	Related Exemplars/Diseases

Reading/Resources - Clinical Judgment	Class/Lab/Clinical – Clinical Judgment

Priority Assessments or Cues	Priority Labs & Diagnostics	Priority Nursing Interventions
1	1	1
2	2	2
3	3	3

Priority Medications	Priority Potential & Actual Complications	Priority Collaborative Goals
1	1	1
2	2	2
3	3	3

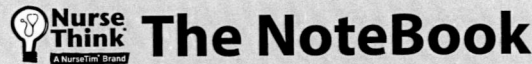
NurseThink® Quick

NEXT GEN LEARNING – NCLEX® TEST PLAN

Safe and Effective Care: Management of Care, Coordinated Care, Safety and Infection Control

Health Promotion and Maintenance

Psychosocial Integrity

Physiological Integrity: Basic Care and Comfort, Pharmacological and Parenteral Therapies, Reduction of Risk Potential, and Physiological Adaptation

QUALITY AND SAFETY COMPETENCIES

Patient-Centered Care

Teamwork and Collaboration

Evidence-Based Practice

Quality Improvement

Safety

Informatics

Peer Review: _____   Faculty Review: _____

Grade Tracker

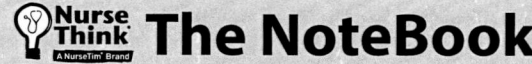 **The NoteBook**

Related Concepts

Related Exemplars/Diseases

Reading/Resources - Clinical Judgment

Class/Lab/Clinical – Clinical Judgment

Priority Assessments or Cues

1

2

3

Priority Labs & Diagnostics

1

2

3

Priority Nursing Interventions

1

2

3

Priority Medications

1

2

3

Priority Potential & Actual Complications

1

2

3

Priority Collaborative Goals

1

2

3

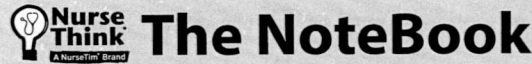
NurseThink® Quick

NEXT GEN LEARNING – NCLEX® TEST PLAN

Safe and Effective Care: Management of Care, Coordinated Care, Safety and Infection Control

Health Promotion and Maintenance

Psychosocial Integrity

Physiological Integrity: Basic Care and Comfort, Pharmacological and Parenteral Therapies, Reduction of Risk Potential, and Physiological Adaptation

QUALITY AND SAFETY COMPETENCIES

Patient-Centered Care

Teamwork and Collaboration

Evidence-Based Practice

Quality Improvement

Safety

Informatics

Peer Review: _____   Faculty Review: _____

Grade Tracker

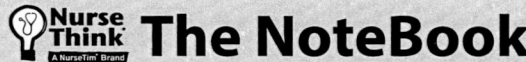

Related Concepts	Related Exemplars/Diseases

Reading/Resources - Clinical Judgment	Class/Lab/Clinical – Clinical Judgment

Priority Assessments or Cues	Priority Labs & Diagnostics	Priority Nursing Interventions
1	1	1
2	2	2
3	3	3

Priority Medications	Priority Potential & Actual Complications	Priority Collaborative Goals
1	1	1
2	2	2
3	3	3

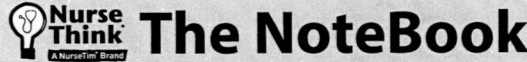

NurseThink® Quick

NEXT GEN LEARNING – NCLEX® TEST PLAN

Safe and Effective Care: Management of Care, Coordinated Care, Safety and Infection Control

Health Promotion and Maintenance

Psychosocial Integrity

Physiological Integrity: Basic Care and Comfort, Pharmacological and Parenteral Therapies, Reduction of Risk Potential, and Physiological Adaptation

QUALITY AND SAFETY COMPETENCIES

Patient-Centered Care

Teamwork and Collaboration

Evidence-Based Practice

Quality Improvement

Safety

Informatics

Peer Review: _____   Faculty Review: _____

Grade Tracker

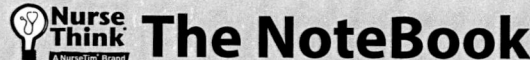

Related Concepts	Related Exemplars/Diseases

Reading/Resources - Clinical Judgment	Class/Lab/Clinical – Clinical Judgment
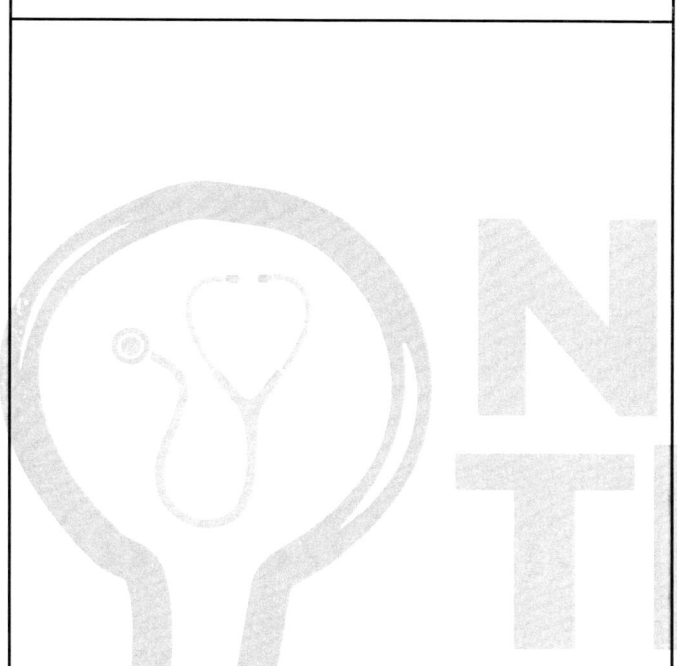	

Priority Assessments or Cues	Priority Labs & Diagnostics	Priority Nursing Interventions
1	1	1
2	2	2
3	3	3

Priority Medications	Priority Potential & Actual Complications	Priority Collaborative Goals
1	1	1
2	2	2
3	3	3

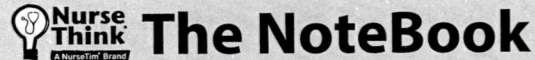
NurseThink® Quick

Pruritus: Systemic Causes

Itch

Iron deficiency anemia/Internal malignancy

Thyroid disease/Type I DM

Chronic renal failure/Chronic liver disease

HIV infection/Hereditary hemochromatosis

NEXT GEN LEARNING – NCLEX® TEST PLAN

Safe and Effective Care: Management of Care, Coordinated Care, Safety and Infection Control

Health Promotion and Maintenance

Psychosocial Integrity

Physiological Integrity: Basic Care and Comfort, Pharmacological and Parenteral Therapies, Reduction of Risk Potential, and Physiological Adaptation

QUALITY AND SAFETY COMPETENCIES

Patient-Centered Care

Teamwork and Collaboration

Evidence-Based Practice

Quality Improvement

Safety

Informatics

Peer Review: _____   Faculty Review: _____

Grade Tracker

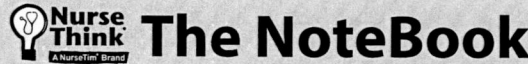

Related Concepts	Related Exemplars/Diseases

Reading/Resources - Clinical Judgment	Class/Lab/Clinical – Clinical Judgment

Priority Assessments or Cues	Priority Labs & Diagnostics	Priority Nursing Interventions
1	1	1
2	2	2
3	3	3

Priority Medications	Priority Potential & Actual Complications	Priority Collaborative Goals
1	1	1
2	2	2
3	3	3

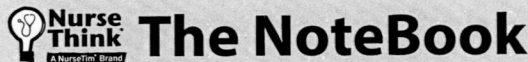
NurseThink® Quick

NEXT GEN LEARNING – NCLEX® TEST PLAN

Safe and Effective Care: Management of Care, Coordinated Care, Safety and Infection Control

Health Promotion and Maintenance

Psychosocial Integrity

Physiological Integrity: Basic Care and Comfort, Pharmacological and Parenteral Therapies, Reduction of Risk Potential, and Physiological Adaptation

QUALITY AND SAFETY COMPETENCIES

Patient-Centered Care

Teamwork and Collaboration

Evidence-Based Practice

Quality Improvement

Safety

Informatics

Peer Review: _____   Faculty Review: _____

Grade Tracker

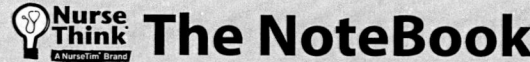

Related Concepts	**Related Exemplars/Diseases**

Reading/Resources - Clinical Judgment	**Class/Lab/Clinical – Clinical Judgment**

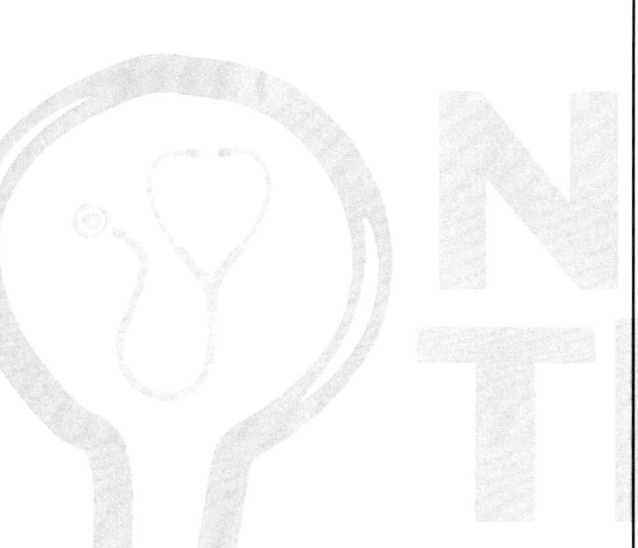

Priority Assessments or Cues	**Priority Labs & Diagnostics**	**Priority Nursing Interventions**
1	1	1
2	2	2
3	3	3

Priority Medications	**Priority Potential & Actual Complications**	**Priority Collaborative Goals**
1	1	1
2	2	2
3	3	3

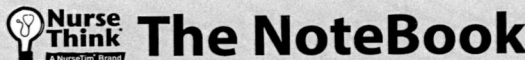
NurseThink® Quick

Pressure Sore: Norton Score

Magic
Mobility
ADL
General condition
Incontinence
Conscious level

NEXT GEN LEARNING – NCLEX® TEST PLAN

Safe and Effective Care: Management of Care, Coordinated Care, Safety and Infection Control

Health Promotion and Maintenance

Psychosocial Integrity

Physiological Integrity: Basic Care and Comfort, Pharmacological and Parenteral Therapies, Reduction of Risk Potential, and Physiological Adaptation

QUALITY AND SAFETY COMPETENCIES

Patient-Centered Care

Teamwork and Collaboration

Evidence-Based Practice

Quality Improvement

Safety

Informatics

Peer Review: _____   Faculty Review: _____

Grade Tracker

Related Concepts

Related Exemplars/Diseases

Reading/Resources - Clinical Judgment

Class/Lab/Clinical – Clinical Judgment

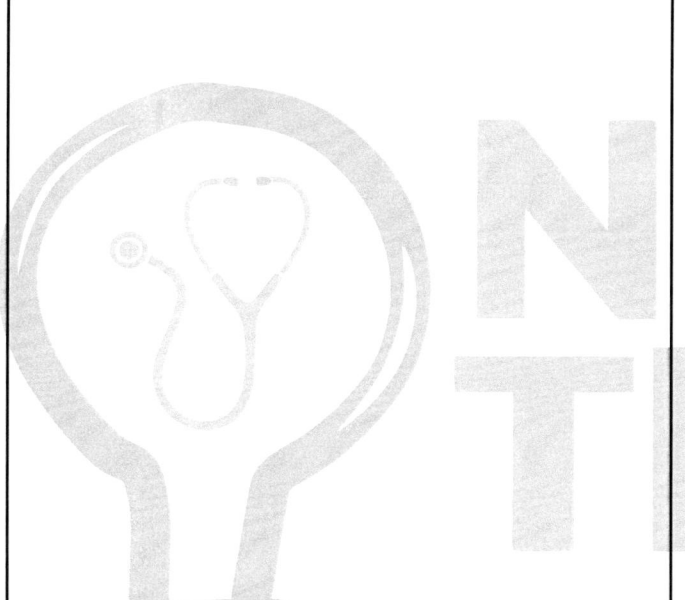

Priority Assessments or Cues	**Priority Labs & Diagnostics**	**Priority Nursing Interventions**
1	1	1
2	2	2
3	3	3

Priority Medications	**Priority Potential & Actual Complications**	**Priority Collaborative Goals**
1	1	1
2	2	2
3	3	3

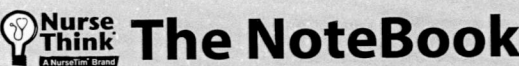
NurseThink® Quick

NEXT GEN LEARNING – NCLEX® TEST PLAN

Safe and Effective Care: Management of Care, Coordinated Care, Safety and Infection Control

Health Promotion and Maintenance

Psychosocial Integrity

Physiological Integrity: Basic Care and Comfort, Pharmacological and Parenteral Therapies, Reduction of Risk Potential, and Physiological Adaptation

QUALITY AND SAFETY COMPETENCIES

Patient-Centered Care

Teamwork and Collaboration

Evidence-Based Practice

Quality Improvement

Safety

Informatics

Peer Review: _____   Faculty Review: _____

Grade Tracker

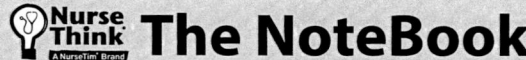
Related Concepts	**Related Exemplars/Diseases**

Reading/Resources - Clinical Judgment	**Class/Lab/Clinical – Clinical Judgment**

Priority Assessments or Cues	**Priority Labs & Diagnostics**	**Priority Nursing Interventions**
1	1	1
2	2	2
3	3	3

Priority Medications	**Priority Potential & Actual Complications**	**Priority Collaborative Goals**
1	1	1
2	2	2
3	3	3

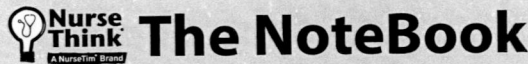
NurseThink® Quick

NEXT GEN LEARNING – NCLEX® TEST PLAN

Safe and Effective Care: Management of Care, Coordinated Care, Safety and Infection Control

Health Promotion and Maintenance

Psychosocial Integrity

Physiological Integrity: Basic Care and Comfort, Pharmacological and Parenteral Therapies, Reduction of Risk Potential, and Physiological Adaptation

QUALITY AND SAFETY COMPETENCIES

Patient-Centered Care

Teamwork and Collaboration

Evidence-Based Practice

Quality Improvement

Safety

Informatics

Peer Review: _____   Faculty Review: _____

Grade Tracker

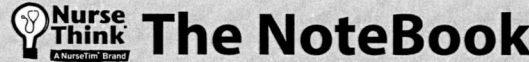
Related Concepts	**Related Exemplars/Diseases**

Reading/Resources - Clinical Judgment	**Class/Lab/Clinical – Clinical Judgment**

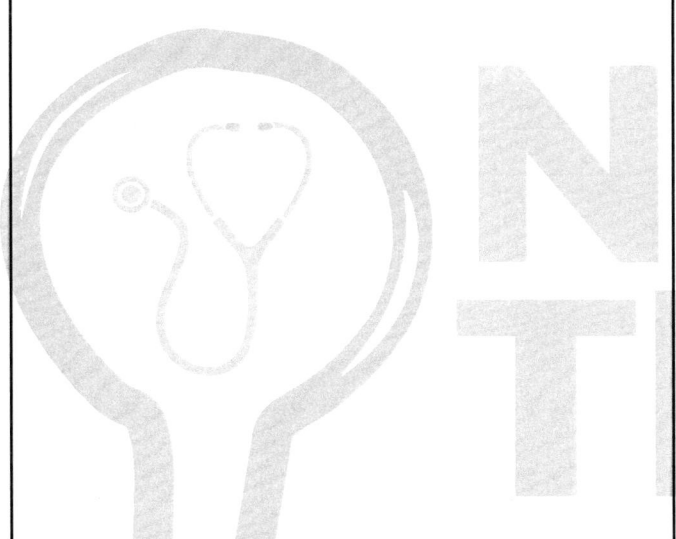

Priority Assessments or Cues	**Priority Labs & Diagnostics**	**Priority Nursing Interventions**
1	1	1
2	2	2
3	3	3

Priority Medications	**Priority Potential & Actual Complications**	**Priority Collaborative Goals**
1	1	1
2	2	2
3	3	3

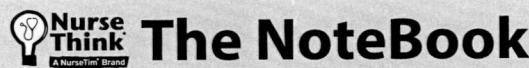
NurseThink® Quick

NEXT GEN LEARNING – NCLEX® TEST PLAN

Safe and Effective Care: Management of Care, Coordinated Care, Safety and Infection Control

Health Promotion and Maintenance

Psychosocial Integrity

Physiological Integrity: Basic Care and Comfort, Pharmacological and Parenteral Therapies, Reduction of Risk Potential, and Physiological Adaptation

QUALITY AND SAFETY COMPETENCIES

Patient-Centered Care

Teamwork and Collaboration

Evidence-Based Practice

Quality Improvement

Safety

Informatics

Peer Review: _____   Faculty Review: _____

Grade Tracker

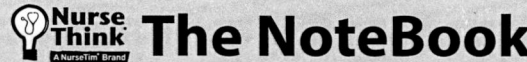
Related Concepts	Related Exemplars/Diseases

Reading/Resources - Clinical Judgment	Class/Lab/Clinical – Clinical Judgment

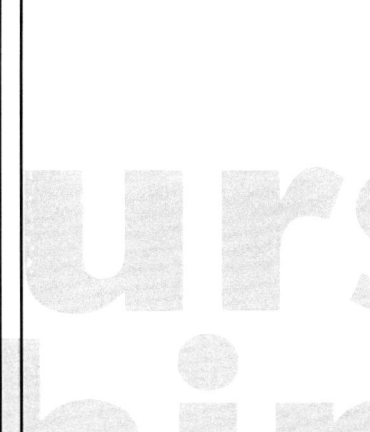
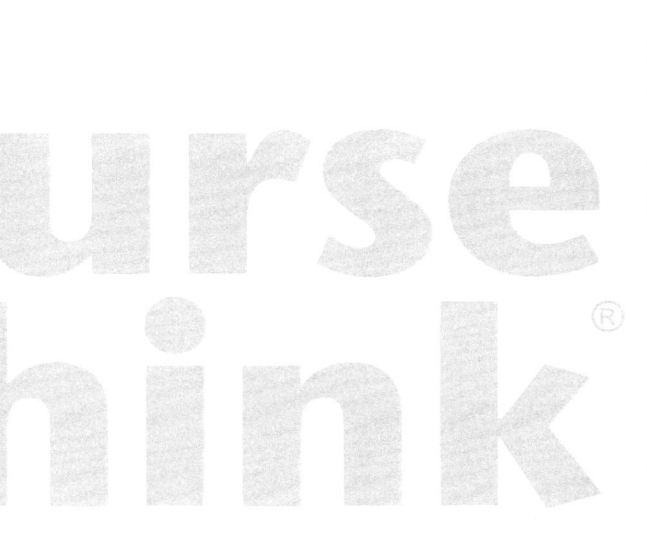

Priority Assessments or Cues	Priority Labs & Diagnostics	Priority Nursing Interventions
1	1	1
2	2	2
3	3	3

Priority Medications	Priority Potential & Actual Complications	Priority Collaborative Goals
1	1	1
2	2	2
3	3	3

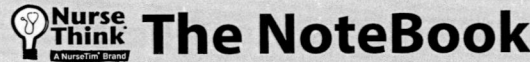
NurseThink® Quick

<table>
<tr><td></td><td></td><td></td></tr>
</table>

NEXT GEN LEARNING – NCLEX® TEST PLAN

Safe and Effective Care: Management of Care, Coordinated Care, Safety and Infection Control

Health Promotion and Maintenance

Psychosocial Integrity

Physiological Integrity: Basic Care and Comfort, Pharmacological and Parenteral Therapies, Reduction of Risk Potential, and Physiological Adaptation

QUALITY AND SAFETY COMPETENCIES

Patient-Centered Care

Teamwork and Collaboration

Evidence-Based Practice

Quality Improvement

Safety

Informatics

Peer Review: _____   Faculty Review: _____

Grade Tracker

<table>
<tr><td></td><td></td><td></td><td></td><td></td><td></td><td></td><td></td><td></td><td></td><td></td><td></td><td></td><td></td><td></td><td></td></tr>
</table>

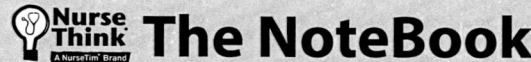
Related Concepts

Related Exemplars/Diseases

Reading/Resources - Clinical Judgment

Class/Lab/Clinical – Clinical Judgment

Priority Assessments or Cues

1

2

3

Priority Labs & Diagnostics

1

2

3

Priority Nursing Interventions

1

2

3

Priority Medications

1

2

3

Priority Potential & Actual Complications

1

2

3

Priority Collaborative Goals

1

2

3

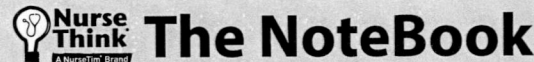
NurseThink® Quick

<table>
<tr><td></td><td></td><td></td></tr>
</table>

NEXT GEN LEARNING – NCLEX® TEST PLAN

Safe and Effective Care: Management of Care, Coordinated Care, Safety and Infection Control

Health Promotion and Maintenance

Psychosocial Integrity

Physiological Integrity: Basic Care and Comfort, Pharmacological and Parenteral Therapies, Reduction of Risk Potential, and Physiological Adaptation

QUALITY AND SAFETY COMPETENCIES

Patient-Centered Care

Teamwork and Collaboration

Evidence-Based Practice

Quality Improvement

Safety

Informatics

Peer Review: _____   Faculty Review: _____

Grade Tracker

<table>
<tr><td></td><td></td><td></td><td></td><td></td><td></td><td></td><td></td><td></td><td></td><td></td><td></td><td></td><td></td><td></td><td></td><td></td></tr>
</table>

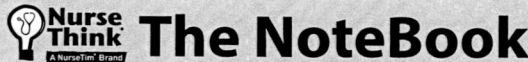
Related Concepts

Related Exemplars/Diseases

Reading/Resources - Clinical Judgment

Class/Lab/Clinical – Clinical Judgment

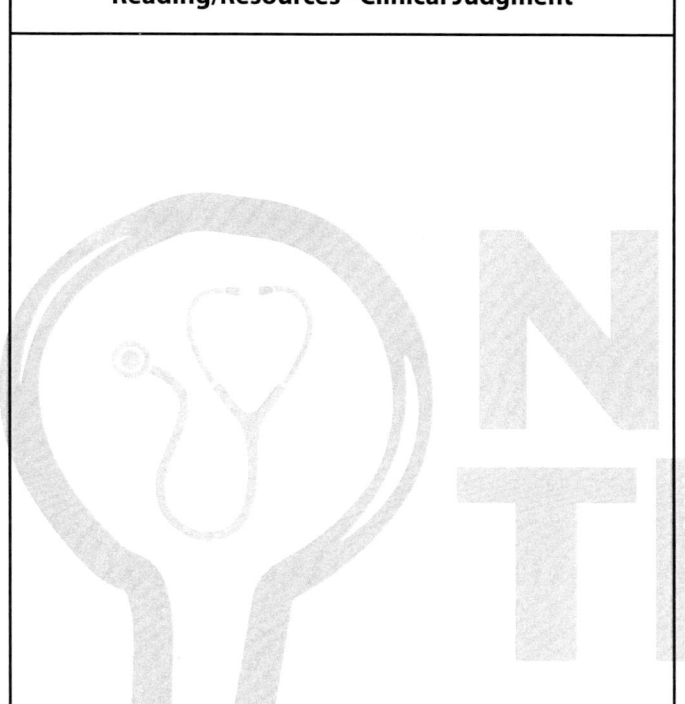

Priority Assessments or Cues

1
2
3

Priority Labs & Diagnostics

1
2
3

Priority Nursing Interventions

1
2
3

Priority Medications

1

2

3

Priority Potential & Actual Complications

1

2

3

Priority Collaborative Goals

1

2

3

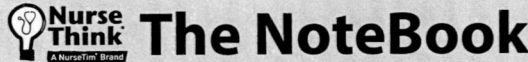
NurseThink® Quick

NEXT GEN LEARNING – NCLEX® TEST PLAN

Safe and Effective Care: Management of Care, Coordinated Care, Safety and Infection Control

Health Promotion and Maintenance

Psychosocial Integrity

Physiological Integrity: Basic Care and Comfort, Pharmacological and Parenteral Therapies, Reduction of Risk Potential, and Physiological Adaptation

QUALITY AND SAFETY COMPETENCIES

Patient-Centered Care

Teamwork and Collaboration

Evidence-Based Practice

Quality Improvement

Safety

Informatics

Peer Review: _____   Faculty Review: _____

Grade Tracker

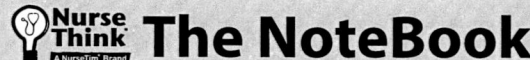

Related Concepts	**Related Exemplars/Diseases**

Reading/Resources - Clinical Judgment	**Class/Lab/Clinical – Clinical Judgment**
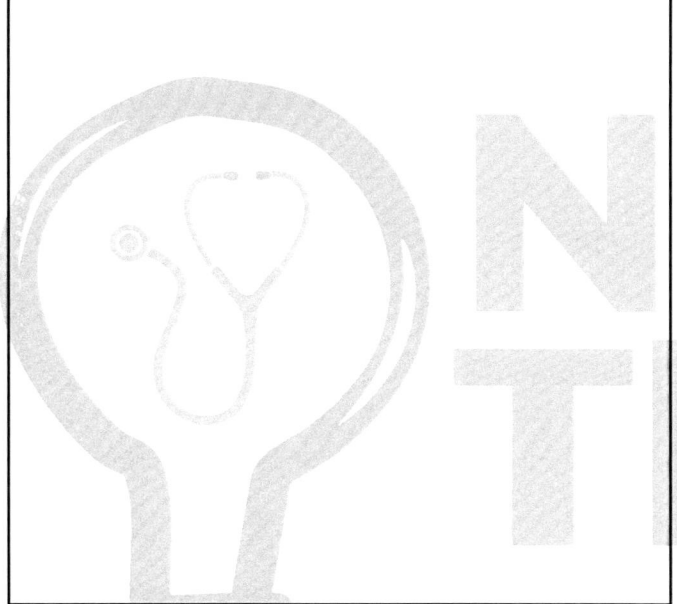	

Priority Assessments or Cues	**Priority Labs & Diagnostics**	**Priority Nursing Interventions**
1	1	1
2	2	2
3	3	3

Priority Medications	**Priority Potential & Actual Complications**	**Priority Collaborative Goals**
1	1	1
2	2	2
3	3	3

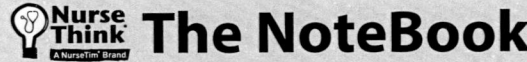
NurseThink® Quick

NEXT GEN LEARNING – NCLEX® TEST PLAN

Safe and Effective Care: Management of Care, Coordinated Care, Safety and Infection Control

Health Promotion and Maintenance

Psychosocial Integrity

Physiological Integrity: Basic Care and Comfort, Pharmacological and Parenteral Therapies, Reduction of Risk Potential, and Physiological Adaptation

QUALITY AND SAFETY COMPETENCIES

Patient-Centered Care

Teamwork and Collaboration

Evidence-Based Practice

Quality Improvement

Safety

Informatics

Peer Review: _____   Faculty Review: _____

Grade Tracker

Related Concepts

Related Exemplars/Diseases

Reading/Resources - Clinical Judgment

Class/Lab/Clinical – Clinical Judgment

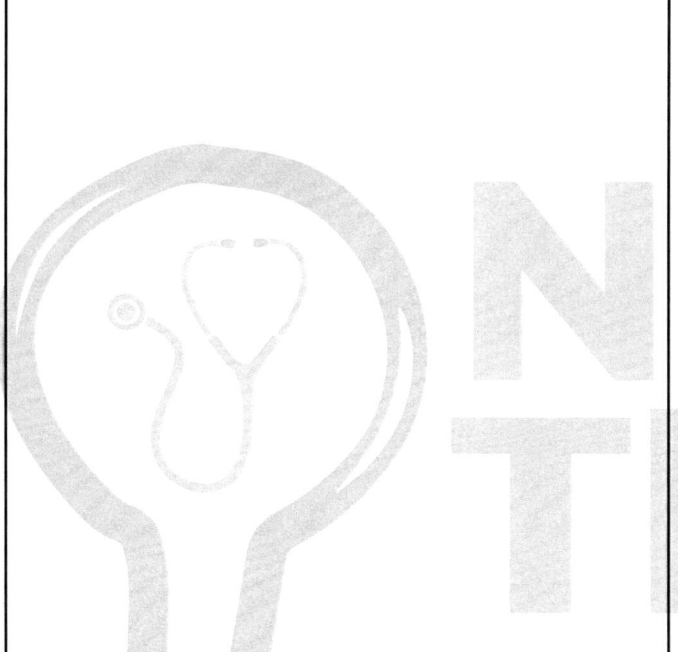

Priority Assessments or Cues

1

2

3

Priority Labs & Diagnostics

1

2

3

Priority Nursing Interventions

1

2

3

Priority Medications

1

2

3

Priority Potential & Actual Complications

1

2

3

Priority Collaborative Goals

1

2

3

NurseThink® Quick

Alkalosis and Acidosis
Alkalosis - has a "k" - kicking the pH up
Acidosis - has a "d" - dropping the pH down

ABG Analysis
Rome
Respiratory
Opposite
Metabolic
Equal

Solutions: Isotonic, Hypotonic, Hypertonic
Isotonic - "same as I" - the solution used will be the same as normal body fluid composition. Fluids remain inside intravascular space.
Hypotonic - "hypo, hippo" - the solution pulls fluid from the intravascular space into the ICF - the cell "swells like a hippo."

Acid-Base Balance
Respiratory: Opposite
ph>7.45 & pco2<35 = respiratory alkalosis
ph<7.35 & pco2>45 = respiratory acidosis
Metabolic: Equal
ph>7.45 & hco3>26 = metabolic alkalosis
ph<7.35 & hco3<22 = metabolic acidosis

NEXT GEN LEARNING – NCLEX® TEST PLAN

Safe and Effective Care: Management of Care, Coordinated Care, Safety and Infection Control

Health Promotion and Maintenance

Psychosocial Integrity

Physiological Integrity: Basic Care and Comfort, Pharmacological and Parenteral Therapies, Reduction of Risk Potential, and Physiological Adaptation

QUALITY AND SAFETY COMPETENCIES

Patient-Centered Care

Teamwork and Collaboration

Evidence-Based Practice

Quality Improvement

Safety

Informatics

Peer Review: _____   Faculty Review: _____

Grade Tracker

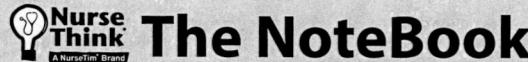

Related Concepts	Related Exemplars/Diseases

Reading/Resources - Clinical Judgment	Class/Lab/Clinical – Clinical Judgment
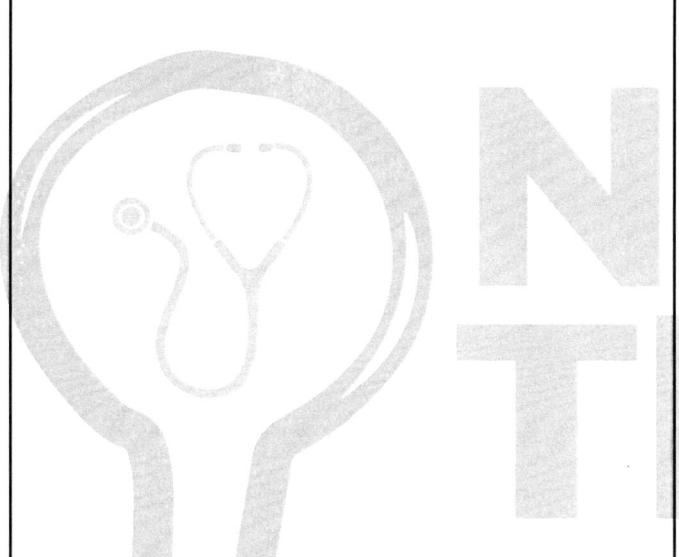	

Priority Assessments or Cues	Priority Labs & Diagnostics	Priority Nursing Interventions
1	1	1
2	2	2
3	3	3

Priority Medications	Priority Potential & Actual Complications	Priority Collaborative Goals
1	1	1
2	2	2
3	3	3

NurseThink® Quick

NEXT GEN LEARNING – NCLEX® TEST PLAN

Safe and Effective Care: Management of Care, Coordinated Care, Safety and Infection Control

Health Promotion and Maintenance

Psychosocial Integrity

Physiological Integrity: Basic Care and Comfort, Pharmacological and Parenteral Therapies, Reduction of Risk Potential, and Physiological Adaptation

QUALITY AND SAFETY COMPETENCIES

Patient-Centered Care

Teamwork and Collaboration

Evidence-Based Practice

Quality Improvement

Safety

Informatics

Peer Review: _____   Faculty Review: _____

Grade Tracker

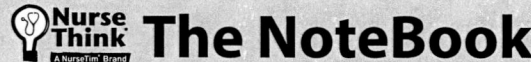
Related Concepts

Related Exemplars/Diseases

Reading/Resources - Clinical Judgment

Class/Lab/Clinical – Clinical Judgment

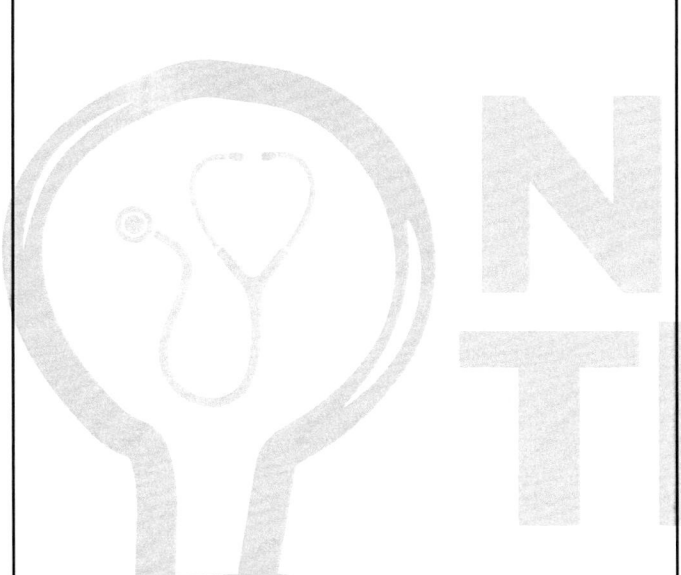

Priority Assessments or Cues

1
2
3

Priority Labs & Diagnostics

1
2
3

Priority Nursing Interventions

1
2
3

Priority Medications

1

2

3

Priority Potential & Actual Complications

1

2

3

Priority Collaborative Goals

1

2

3

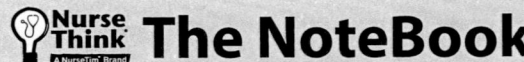

NurseThink® Quick

<table>
<tr><td></td><td></td><td></td></tr>
</table>

NEXT GEN LEARNING – NCLEX® TEST PLAN

Safe and Effective Care: Management of Care, Coordinated Care, Safety and Infection Control

Health Promotion and Maintenance

Psychosocial Integrity

Physiological Integrity: Basic Care and Comfort, Pharmacological and Parenteral Therapies, Reduction of Risk Potential, and Physiological Adaptation

QUALITY AND SAFETY COMPETENCIES

Patient-Centered Care

Teamwork and Collaboration

Evidence-Based Practice

Quality Improvement

Safety

Informatics

Peer Review: _____   Faculty Review: _____

Grade Tracker

<table>
<tr><td></td><td></td><td></td><td></td><td></td><td></td><td></td><td></td><td></td><td></td><td></td><td></td><td></td><td></td><td></td><td></td></tr>
</table>

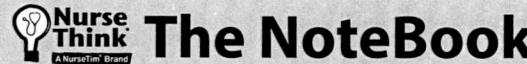
Related Concepts	**Related Exemplars/Diseases**

Reading/Resources - Clinical Judgment	**Class/Lab/Clinical – Clinical Judgment**

Priority Assessments or Cues	**Priority Labs & Diagnostics**	**Priority Nursing Interventions**
1	1	1
2	2	2
3	3	3

Priority Medications	**Priority Potential & Actual Complications**	**Priority Collaborative Goals**
1	1	1
2	2	2
3	3	3

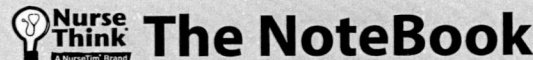
NurseThink® Quick

NEXT GEN LEARNING – NCLEX® TEST PLAN

Safe and Effective Care: Management of Care, Coordinated Care, Safety and Infection Control

Health Promotion and Maintenance

Psychosocial Integrity

Physiological Integrity: Basic Care and Comfort, Pharmacological and Parenteral Therapies, Reduction of Risk Potential, and Physiological Adaptation

QUALITY AND SAFETY COMPETENCIES

Patient-Centered Care

Teamwork and Collaboration

Evidence-Based Practice

Quality Improvement

Safety

Informatics

Peer Review: _____   Faculty Review: _____

Grade Tracker

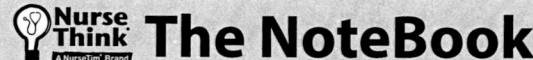
Related Concepts	**Related Exemplars/Diseases**

Reading/Resources - Clinical Judgment	**Class/Lab/Clinical – Clinical Judgment**

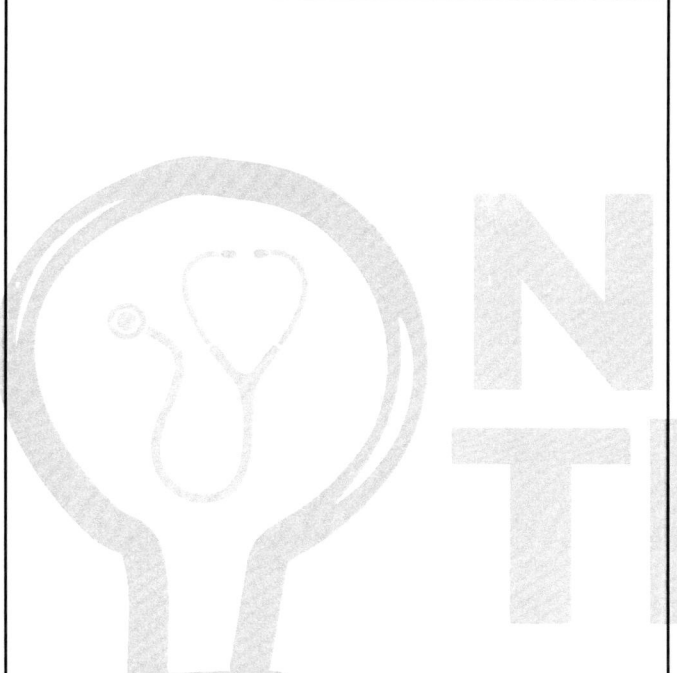

Priority Assessments or Cues	**Priority Labs & Diagnostics**	**Priority Nursing Interventions**
1	1	1
2	2	2
3	3	3

Priority Medications	**Priority Potential & Actual Complications**	**Priority Collaborative Goals**
1	1	1
2	2	2
3	3	3

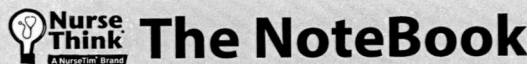
NurseThink® Quick

NEXT GEN LEARNING – NCLEX® TEST PLAN

Safe and Effective Care: Management of Care, Coordinated Care, Safety and Infection Control

Health Promotion and Maintenance

Psychosocial Integrity

Physiological Integrity: Basic Care and Comfort, Pharmacological and Parenteral Therapies, Reduction of Risk Potential, and Physiological Adaptation

QUALITY AND SAFETY COMPETENCIES

Patient-Centered Care

Teamwork and Collaboration

Evidence-Based Practice

Quality Improvement

Safety

Informatics

Peer Review: _____   Faculty Review: _____

Grade Tracker

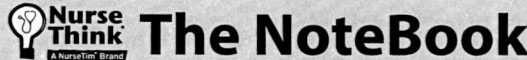

Related Concepts	Related Exemplars/Diseases

Reading/Resources - Clinical Judgment	Class/Lab/Clinical – Clinical Judgment

Priority Assessments or Cues	Priority Labs & Diagnostics	Priority Nursing Interventions
1	1	1
2	2	2
3	3	3

Priority Medications	Priority Potential & Actual Complications	Priority Collaborative Goals
1	1	1
2	2	2
3	3	3

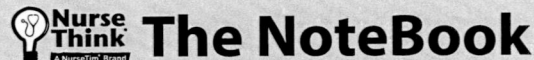
NurseThink® Quick

Hypercalcemia: Signs and Symptoms	**Hypercalcemia: Causes**	**Hypocalcemia: Signs and Symptoms**
Groans, Moans, Bones, Stones, and Overtones	*MD Pimps Me*	*Cats*
Groans: constipation	**M**alignancy	**C**onvulsions
Moans: pain - joint aches	**D**iuretics	**A**rrhythmias
Bones: loss of calcium from bones, bone metastasis	**P**arathyroid	**T**etany
Stones: kidney stones	**I**mmobilization/ Idiopathic	**S**pasms and stridor
Overtones: psychiatric overtones - depression, confusion	**M**ega doses of vitamins A, D P – Paget's Disease	
	Sarcoidosis	
	Milk alkali syndrome	
	Endocrine (Addison's disease, thyrotoxicosis)	

NEXT GEN LEARNING – NCLEX® TEST PLAN

Safe and Effective Care: Management of Care, Coordinated Care, Safety and Infection Control

Health Promotion and Maintenance

Psychosocial Integrity

Physiological Integrity: Basic Care and Comfort, Pharmacological and Parenteral Therapies, Reduction of Risk Potential, and Physiological Adaptation

QUALITY AND SAFETY COMPETENCIES

Patient-Centered Care

Teamwork and Collaboration

Evidence-Based Practice

Quality Improvement

Safety

Informatics

Peer Review: _____ Faculty Review: _____

Grade Tracker

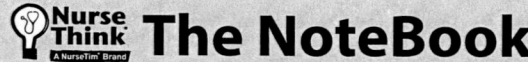
Related Concepts

Related Exemplars/Diseases

Reading/Resources - Clinical Judgment

Class/Lab/Clinical – Clinical Judgment

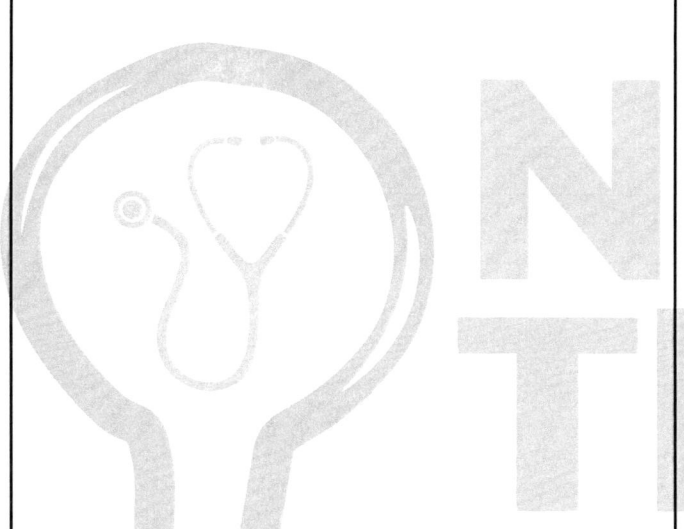

Priority Assessments or Cues

1

2

3

Priority Labs & Diagnostics

1

2

3

Priority Nursing Interventions

1

2

3

Priority Medications

1

2

3

Priority Potential & Actual Complications

1

2

3

Priority Collaborative Goals

1

2

3

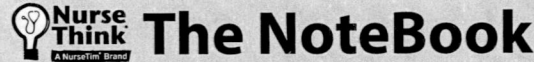
NurseThink® Quick

Hyperkalemia: Causes
Machine
Medications - ACE inhibitors, NSAIDS
Acidosis - metabolic and respiratory
Cellular destruction - burns, traumatic injury
Hypoaldosteronism, hemolysis
Intake - excessive
Nephrons, renal failure
Excretion – impaired

Hyperkalemia: Signs and Symptoms
Murder
Muscle weakness
Urine, oliguria, anuria
Respiratory distress
Decreased cardiac contractility
ECG changes
Reflexes, hyperreflexia, or areflexia (flaccid)

Hyperkalemia: Treatment
Kind
Kayexalate
Insulin
Na HCO3
Diuretics

Hypokalemia: Signs and Symptoms
6 L's
Lethargy
Leg cramps
Limp muscles
Low, shallow respirations
Lethal cardiac dysrhythmias
Lots of urine (polyuria)

NEXT GEN LEARNING – NCLEX® TEST PLAN

Safe and Effective Care: Management of Care, Coordinated Care, Safety and Infection Control

Health Promotion and Maintenance

Psychosocial Integrity

Physiological Integrity: Basic Care and Comfort, Pharmacological and Parenteral Therapies, Reduction of Risk Potential, and Physiological Adaptation

QUALITY AND SAFETY COMPETENCIES

Patient-Centered Care

Teamwork and Collaboration

Evidence-Based Practice

Quality Improvement

Safety

Informatics

Peer Review: _____   Faculty Review: _____

Grade Tracker

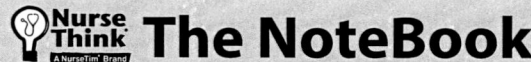

Related Concepts

Related Exemplars/Diseases

Reading/Resources - Clinical Judgment

Class/Lab/Clinical – Clinical Judgment

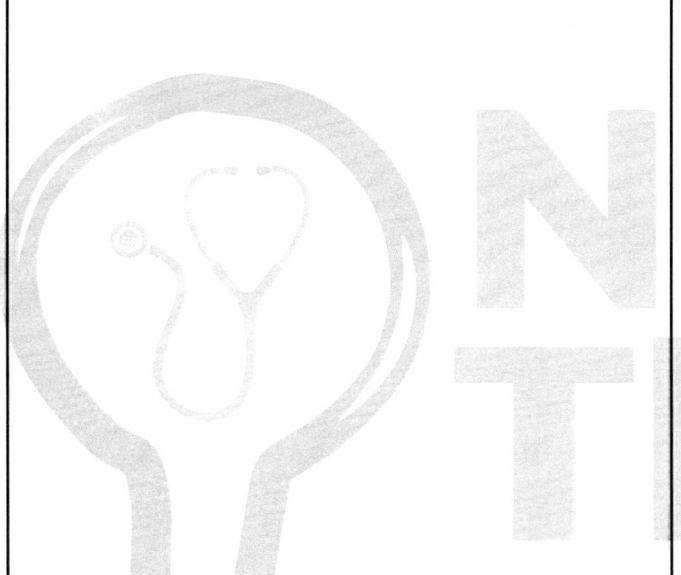

Priority Assessments or Cues

1

2

3

Priority Labs & Diagnostics

1

2

3

Priority Nursing Interventions

1

2

3

Priority Medications

1

2

3

Priority Potential & Actual Complications

1

2

3

Priority Collaborative Goals

1

2

3

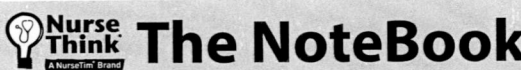
NurseThink® Quick

NEXT GEN LEARNING – NCLEX® TEST PLAN

Safe and Effective Care: Management of Care, Coordinated Care, Safety and Infection Control

Health Promotion and Maintenance

Psychosocial Integrity

Physiological Integrity: Basic Care and Comfort, Pharmacological and Parenteral Therapies, Reduction of Risk Potential, and Physiological Adaptation

QUALITY AND SAFETY COMPETENCIES

Patient-Centered Care

Teamwork and Collaboration

Evidence-Based Practice

Quality Improvement

Safety

Informatics

Peer Review: _____   Faculty Review: _____

Grade Tracker

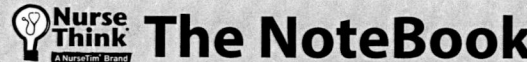
Related Concepts	**Related Exemplars/Diseases**

Reading/Resources - Clinical Judgment	**Class/Lab/Clinical – Clinical Judgment**

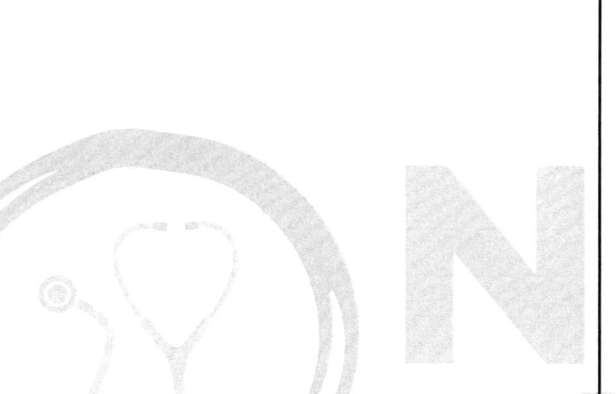

Priority Assessments or Cues	**Priority Labs & Diagnostics**	**Priority Nursing Interventions**
1	1	1
2	2	2
3	3	3

Priority Medications	**Priority Potential & Actual Complications**	**Priority Collaborative Goals**
1	1	1
2	2	2
3	3	3

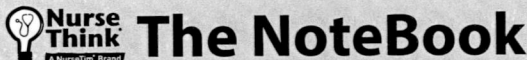
NurseThink® Quick

Hypernatremia: Causes
Model
Medications, meals
Osmotic diuretics
Diabetes insipidus
Excessive water loss
Low water intake

Hypernatremia: Signs and Symptoms
Fried
Fever (low grade), flushed skin
Restless and irritable
Increased fluid retention and increased BP
Edema (peripheral and pitting)
Decreased urinary output, dry mouth

Hyponatremia: Signs and Symptoms
Salt Loss
Stupor and coma
Anorexia, N&V
Lethargy
Tendon reflexes decreased
Limp muscles (weakness)
Orthostatic hypotension
Seizures and headaches
Stomach cramping

NEXT GEN LEARNING – NCLEX® TEST PLAN

Safe and Effective Care: Management of Care, Coordinated Care, Safety and Infection Control

Health Promotion and Maintenance

Psychosocial Integrity

Physiological Integrity: Basic Care and Comfort, Pharmacological and Parenteral Therapies, Reduction of Risk Potential, and Physiological Adaptation

QUALITY AND SAFETY COMPETENCIES

Patient-Centered Care

Teamwork and Collaboration

Evidence-Based Practice

Quality Improvement

Safety

Informatics

Peer Review: _____   Faculty Review: _____

Grade Tracker

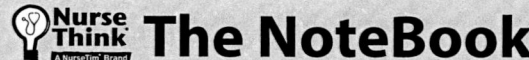

Related Concepts	Related Exemplars/Diseases

Reading/Resources - Clinical Judgment	Class/Lab/Clinical – Clinical Judgment

Priority Assessments or Cues	Priority Labs & Diagnostics	Priority Nursing Interventions
1	1	1
2	2	2
3	3	3

Priority Medications	Priority Potential & Actual Complications	Priority Collaborative Goals
1	1	1
2	2	2
3	3	3

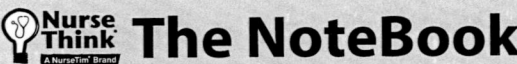
NurseThink® Quick

NEXT GEN LEARNING – NCLEX® TEST PLAN

Safe and Effective Care: Management of Care, Coordinated Care, Safety and Infection Control

Health Promotion and Maintenance

Psychosocial Integrity

Physiological Integrity: Basic Care and Comfort, Pharmacological and Parenteral Therapies, Reduction of Risk Potential, and Physiological Adaptation

QUALITY AND SAFETY COMPETENCIES

Patient-Centered Care

Teamwork and Collaboration

Evidence-Based Practice

Quality Improvement

Safety

Informatics

Peer Review: _____   Faculty Review: _____

Grade Tracker

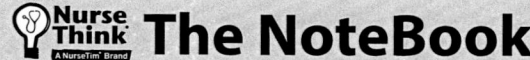

Related Concepts

Related Exemplars/Diseases

Reading/Resources - Clinical Judgment

Class/Lab/Clinical – Clinical Judgment

Priority Assessments or Cues

1

2

3

Priority Labs & Diagnostics

1

2

3

Priority Nursing Interventions

1

2

3

Priority Medications

1

2

3

Priority Potential & Actual Complications

1

2

3

Priority Collaborative Goals

1

2

3

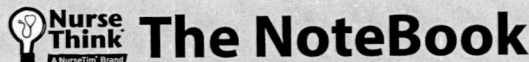
NurseThink® Quick

NEXT GEN LEARNING – NCLEX® TEST PLAN

Safe and Effective Care: Management of Care, Coordinated Care, Safety and Infection Control

Health Promotion and Maintenance

Psychosocial Integrity

Physiological Integrity: Basic Care and Comfort, Pharmacological and Parenteral Therapies, Reduction of Risk Potential, and Physiological Adaptation

QUALITY AND SAFETY COMPETENCIES

Patient-Centered Care

Teamwork and Collaboration

Evidence-Based Practice

Quality Improvement

Safety

Informatics

Peer Review: _____ Faculty Review: _____

Grade Tracker

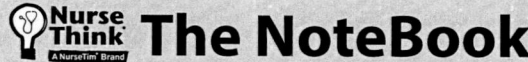

Related Concepts	Related Exemplars/Diseases

Reading/Resources - Clinical Judgment	Class/Lab/Clinical – Clinical Judgment

Priority Assessments or Cues	Priority Labs & Diagnostics	Priority Nursing Interventions
1	1	1
2	2	2
3	3	3

Priority Medications	Priority Potential & Actual Complications	Priority Collaborative Goals
1	1	1
2	2	2
3	3	3

NurseThink® Quick

NEXT GEN LEARNING – NCLEX® TEST PLAN

Safe and Effective Care: Management of Care, Coordinated Care, Safety and Infection Control

Health Promotion and Maintenance

Psychosocial Integrity

Physiological Integrity: Basic Care and Comfort, Pharmacological and Parenteral Therapies, Reduction of Risk Potential, and Physiological Adaptation

QUALITY AND SAFETY COMPETENCIES

Patient-Centered Care

Teamwork and Collaboration

Evidence-Based Practice

Quality Improvement

Safety

Informatics

Peer Review: _____   Faculty Review: _____

Grade Tracker

Related Concepts

Related Exemplars/Diseases

Reading/Resources - Clinical Judgment

Class/Lab/Clinical – Clinical Judgment

Priority Assessments or Cues
1
2
3

Priority Labs & Diagnostics
1
2
3

Priority Nursing Interventions
1
2
3

Priority Medications
1
2
3

Priority Potential & Actual Complications
1
2
3

Priority Collaborative Goals
1
2
3

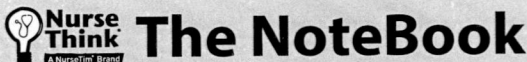
NurseThink® Quick

Assistive devices: Canes		
Coal **C**ane **O**pposite **A**ffected **L**eg		

NEXT GEN LEARNING – NCLEX® TEST PLAN

Safe and Effective Care: Management of Care, Coordinated Care, Safety and Infection Control

Health Promotion and Maintenance

Psychosocial Integrity

Physiological Integrity: Basic Care and Comfort, Pharmacological and Parenteral Therapies, Reduction of Risk Potential, and Physiological Adaptation

QUALITY AND SAFETY COMPETENCIES

Patient-Centered Care

Teamwork and Collaboration

Evidence-Based Practice

Quality Improvement

Safety

Informatics

Peer Review: _____   Faculty Review: _____

Grade Tracker

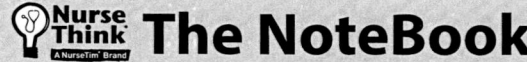

The NoteBook

Related Concepts

Related Exemplars/Diseases

Reading/Resources - Clinical Judgment

Class/Lab/Clinical – Clinical Judgment

Priority Assessments or Cues
1
2
3

Priority Labs & Diagnostics
1
2
3

Priority Nursing Interventions
1
2
3

Priority Medications
1

2

3

Priority Potential & Actual Complications
1

2

3

Priority Collaborative Goals
1

2

3

NurseThink® Quick

NEXT GEN LEARNING – NCLEX® TEST PLAN

Safe and Effective Care: Management of Care, Coordinated Care, Safety and Infection Control

Health Promotion and Maintenance

Psychosocial Integrity

Physiological Integrity: Basic Care and Comfort, Pharmacological and Parenteral Therapies, Reduction of Risk Potential, and Physiological Adaptation

QUALITY AND SAFETY COMPETENCIES

Patient-Centered Care

Teamwork and Collaboration

Evidence-Based Practice

Quality Improvement

Safety

Informatics

Peer Review: _____   Faculty Review: _____

Grade Tracker

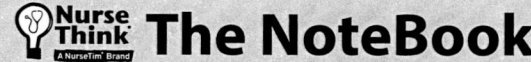
Related Concepts

Related Exemplars/Diseases

Reading/Resources - Clinical Judgment

Class/Lab/Clinical – Clinical Judgment

Priority Assessments or Cues

1

2

3

Priority Labs & Diagnostics

1

2

3

Priority Nursing Interventions

1

2

3

Priority Medications

1

2

3

Priority Potential & Actual Complications

1

2

3

Priority Collaborative Goals

1

2

3

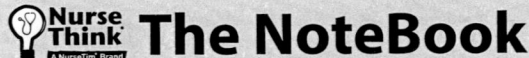
NurseThink® Quick

Carpal Tunnel Syndrome	Carpal Tunnel Treatment	
Dog Arm Pit	***Wrist***	
Dialysis	**W**ear splints at night	
Obesity	**R**est	
Gout	**I**nject steroid	
Amyloid/Acromegaly	**S**urgical decompression	
Rheumatoid arthritis	**T**ake diuretics	
Myxedema		
Pregnancy		
Idiopathic		
Trauma		

NEXT GEN LEARNING – NCLEX® TEST PLAN

Safe and Effective Care: Management of Care, Coordinated Care, Safety and Infection Control

Health Promotion and Maintenance

Psychosocial Integrity

Physiological Integrity: Basic Care and Comfort, Pharmacological and Parenteral Therapies, Reduction of Risk Potential, and Physiological Adaptation

QUALITY AND SAFETY COMPETENCIES

Patient-Centered Care

Teamwork and Collaboration

Evidence-Based Practice

Quality Improvement

Safety

Informatics

Peer Review: _____   Faculty Review: _____

Grade Tracker

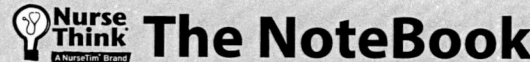

Related Concepts	Related Exemplars/Diseases

Reading/Resources - Clinical Judgment	Class/Lab/Clinical – Clinical Judgment

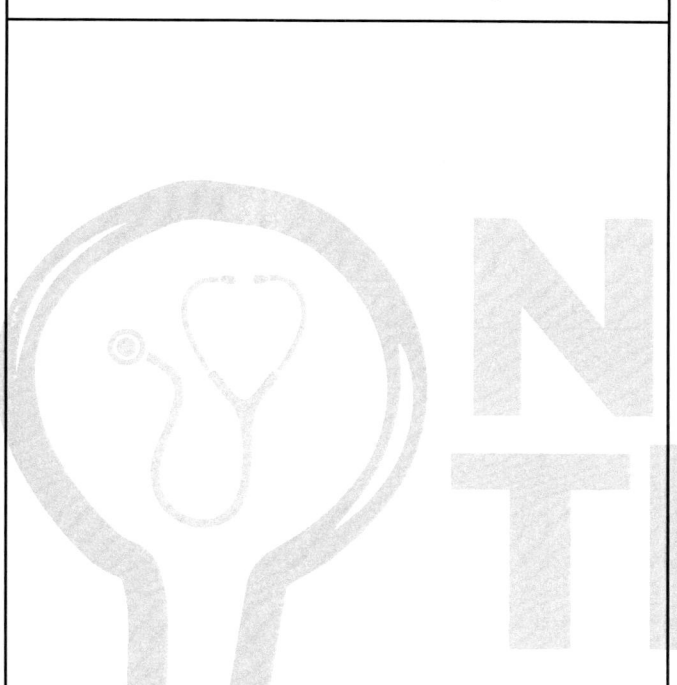

Priority Assessments or Cues	Priority Labs & Diagnostics	Priority Nursing Interventions
1	1	1
2	2	2
3	3	3

Priority Medications	Priority Potential & Actual Complications	Priority Collaborative Goals
1	1	1
2	2	2
3	3	3

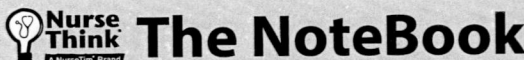
NurseThink® Quick

Fracture: Description
Doctor
Displaced vs. non-displaced
Open vs. closed
Complete vs. incomplete
Transverse vs. linear
Open
Reduction vs. closed reduction

Fractures: Management
Friar
First Aid
Reduction
Immobilization
Active
Rehabilitation

Fractures: Types
Go C3PO
Greenstick
Open
Complete/Closed/Comminuted
Partial
Others

Fracture: Description
BLT Lard
Bone
Location on bone
Type of fracture
Lengthening
Angulation
Rotation
Displacement

NEXT GEN LEARNING – NCLEX® TEST PLAN

Safe and Effective Care: Management of Care, Coordinated Care, Safety and Infection Control

Health Promotion and Maintenance

Psychosocial Integrity

Physiological Integrity: Basic Care and Comfort, Pharmacological and Parenteral Therapies, Reduction of Risk Potential, and Physiological Adaptation

---

QUALITY AND SAFETY COMPETENCIES

Patient-Centered Care

Teamwork and Collaboration

Evidence-Based Practice

Quality Improvement

Safety

Informatics

Peer Review: _____   Faculty Review: _____

Grade Tracker

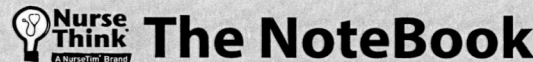
Related Concepts	**Related Exemplars/Diseases**

Reading/Resources - Clinical Judgment	**Class/Lab/Clinical – Clinical Judgment**

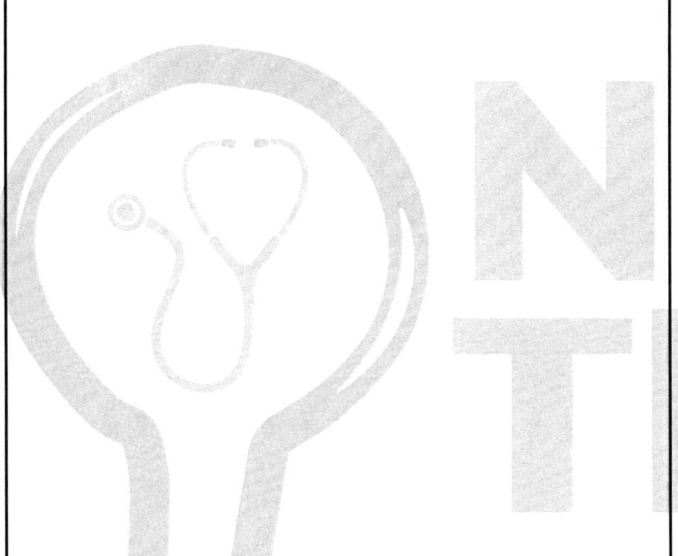

Priority Assessments or Cues	**Priority Labs & Diagnostics**	**Priority Nursing Interventions**
1	1	1
2	2	2
3	3	3

Priority Medications	**Priority Potential & Actual Complications**	**Priority Collaborative Goals**
1	1	1
2	2	2
3	3	3

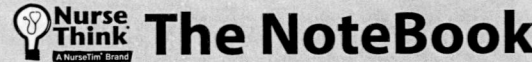
NurseThink® Quick

<table>
<tr><td></td><td></td><td></td></tr>
</table>

NEXT GEN LEARNING – NCLEX® TEST PLAN

Safe and Effective Care: Management of Care, Coordinated Care, Safety and Infection Control

Health Promotion and Maintenance

Psychosocial Integrity

Physiological Integrity: Basic Care and Comfort, Pharmacological and Parenteral Therapies, Reduction of Risk Potential, and Physiological Adaptation

QUALITY AND SAFETY COMPETENCIES

Patient-Centered Care

Teamwork and Collaboration

Evidence-Based Practice

Quality Improvement

Safety

Informatics

Peer Review: _____   Faculty Review: _____

Grade Tracker

<table>
<tr><td></td><td></td><td></td><td></td><td></td><td></td><td></td><td></td><td></td><td></td><td></td><td></td><td></td><td></td><td></td><td></td></tr>
</table>

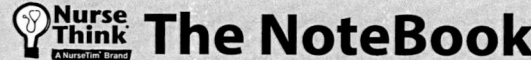
Related Concepts	Related Exemplars/Diseases

Reading/Resources - Clinical Judgment	Class/Lab/Clinical – Clinical Judgment
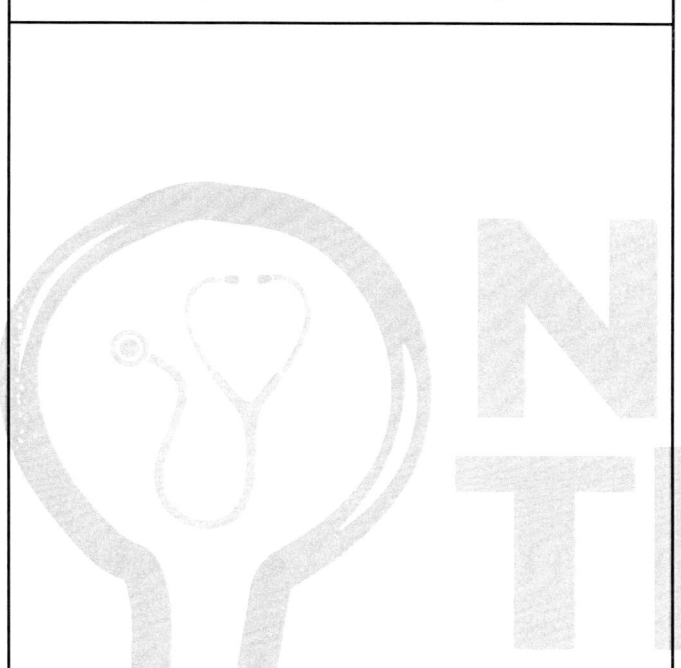	

Priority Assessments or Cues	Priority Labs & Diagnostics	Priority Nursing Interventions
1	1	1
2	2	2
3	3	3

Priority Medications	Priority Potential & Actual Complications	Priority Collaborative Goals
1	1	1
2	2	2
3	3	3

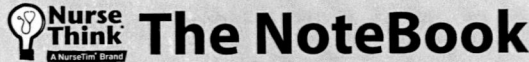
NurseThink® Quick

NEXT GEN LEARNING – NCLEX® TEST PLAN

Safe and Effective Care: Management of Care, Coordinated Care, Safety and Infection Control

Health Promotion and Maintenance

Psychosocial Integrity

Physiological Integrity: Basic Care and Comfort, Pharmacological and Parenteral Therapies, Reduction of Risk Potential, and Physiological Adaptation

QUALITY AND SAFETY COMPETENCIES

Patient-Centered Care

Teamwork and Collaboration

Evidence-Based Practice

Quality Improvement

Safety

Informatics

Peer Review: _____   Faculty Review: _____

Grade Tracker

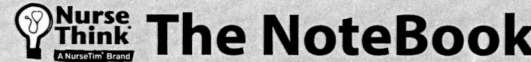
Related Concepts	Related Exemplars/Diseases

Reading/Resources - Clinical Judgment	Class/Lab/Clinical – Clinical Judgment

Priority Assessments or Cues	Priority Labs & Diagnostics	Priority Nursing Interventions
1	1	1
2	2	2
3	3	3

Priority Medications	Priority Potential & Actual Complications	Priority Collaborative Goals
1	1	1
2	2	2
3	3	3

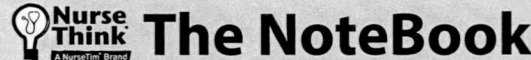
NurseThink® Quick

Restless Leg Syndrome: Symptoms		
Urge **U**rge or sensation to move the legs **R**est or stillness of the legs worsens the urge to move **G**oing is good **E**vening or nighttime worsening of symptoms		

NEXT GEN LEARNING – NCLEX® TEST PLAN

Safe and Effective Care: Management of Care, Coordinated Care, Safety and Infection Control

Health Promotion and Maintenance

Psychosocial Integrity

Physiological Integrity: Basic Care and Comfort, Pharmacological and Parenteral Therapies, Reduction of Risk Potential, and Physiological Adaptation

QUALITY AND SAFETY COMPETENCIES

Patient-Centered Care

Teamwork and Collaboration

Evidence-Based Practice

Quality Improvement

Safety

Informatics

Peer Review: _____   Faculty Review: _____

Grade Tracker

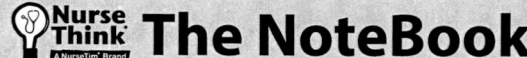
Related Concepts	Related Exemplars/Diseases

Reading/Resources - Clinical Judgment	Class/Lab/Clinical – Clinical Judgment

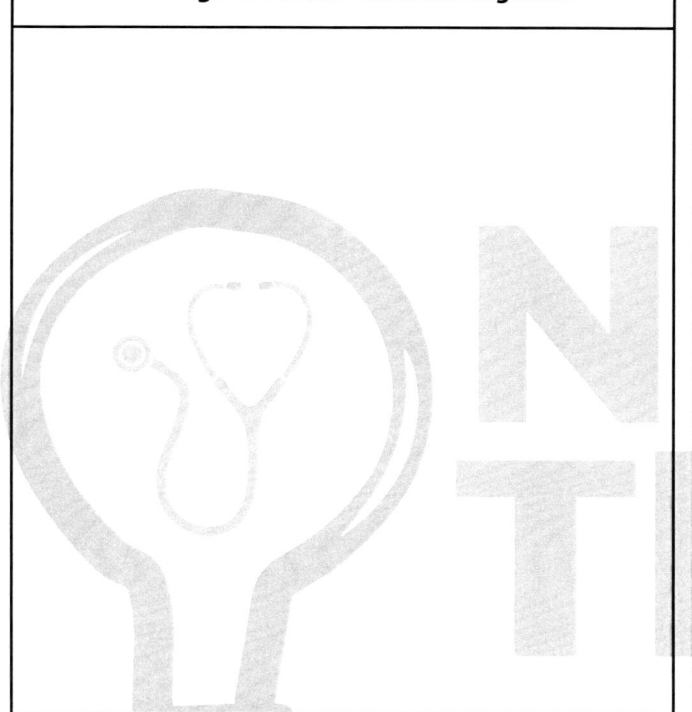

Priority Assessments or Cues

1

2

3

Priority Labs & Diagnostics

1

2

3

Priority Nursing Interventions

1

2

3

Priority Medications

1

2

3

Priority Potential & Actual Complications

1

2

3

Priority Collaborative Goals

1

2

3

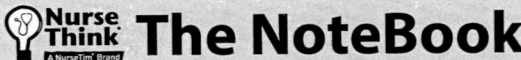
NurseThink® Quick

ALS: Symptoms		
ALS **A**nterior horn neuron loss **L**ower motor dominant effects **S**pino-cortical tract		

NEXT GEN LEARNING – NCLEX® TEST PLAN

Safe and Effective Care: Management of Care, Coordinated Care, Safety and Infection Control

Health Promotion and Maintenance

Psychosocial Integrity

Physiological Integrity: Basic Care and Comfort, Pharmacological and Parenteral Therapies, Reduction of Risk Potential, and Physiological Adaptation

QUALITY AND SAFETY COMPETENCIES

Patient-Centered Care

Teamwork and Collaboration

Evidence-Based Practice

Quality Improvement

Safety

Informatics

Peer Review: _____   Faculty Review: _____

Grade Tracker

Related Concepts	**Related Exemplars/Diseases**

Reading/Resources - Clinical Judgment	**Class/Lab/Clinical – Clinical Judgment**

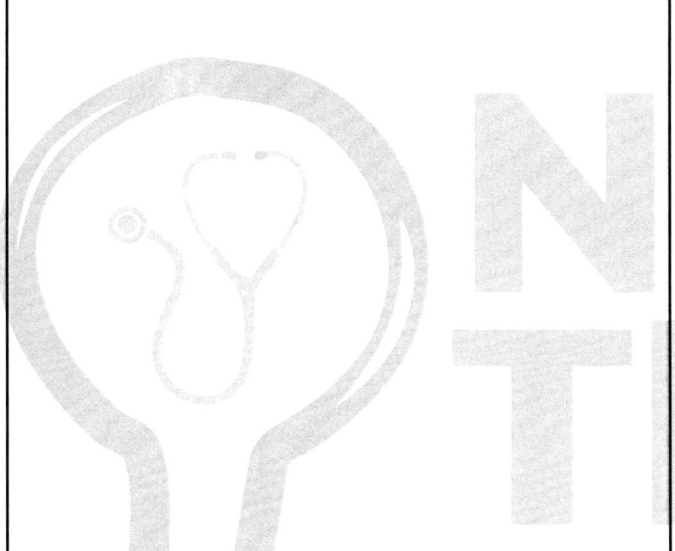

Priority Assessments or Cues	**Priority Labs & Diagnostics**	**Priority Nursing Interventions**
1	1	1
2	2	2
3	3	3

Priority Medications	**Priority Potential & Actual Complications**	**Priority Collaborative Goals**
1	1	1
2	2	2
3	3	3

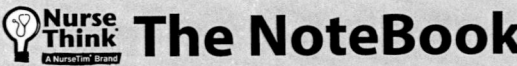

NurseThink® Quick

NEXT GEN LEARNING – NCLEX® TEST PLAN

Safe and Effective Care: Management of Care, Coordinated Care, Safety and Infection Control

Health Promotion and Maintenance

Psychosocial Integrity

Physiological Integrity: Basic Care and Comfort, Pharmacological and Parenteral Therapies, Reduction of Risk Potential, and Physiological Adaptation

QUALITY AND SAFETY COMPETENCIES

Patient-Centered Care

Teamwork and Collaboration

Evidence-Based Practice

Quality Improvement

Safety

Informatics

Peer Review: _____   Faculty Review: _____

Grade Tracker

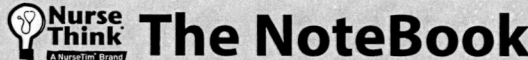
Related Concepts	Related Exemplars/Diseases

Reading/Resources - Clinical Judgment	Class/Lab/Clinical – Clinical Judgment
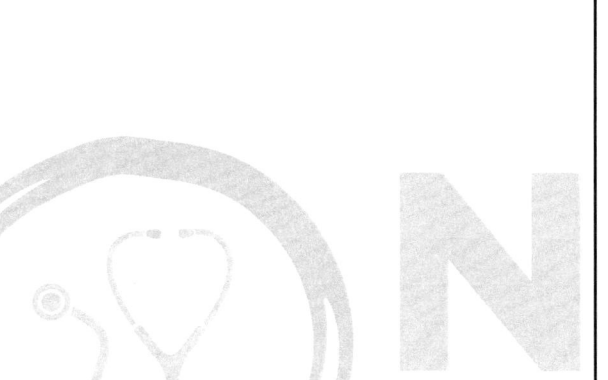	

Priority Assessments or Cues	Priority Labs & Diagnostics	Priority Nursing Interventions
1	1	1
2	2	2
3	3	3

Priority Medications	Priority Potential & Actual Complications	Priority Collaborative Goals
1	1	1
2	2	2
3	3	3

NurseThink® Quick

<table>
<tr><td></td><td></td><td></td></tr>
</table>

NEXT GEN LEARNING – NCLEX® TEST PLAN

Safe and Effective Care: Management of Care, Coordinated Care, Safety and Infection Control

Health Promotion and Maintenance

Psychosocial Integrity

Physiological Integrity: Basic Care and Comfort, Pharmacological and Parenteral Therapies, Reduction of Risk Potential, and Physiological Adaptation

QUALITY AND SAFETY COMPETENCIES

Patient-Centered Care

Teamwork and Collaboration

Evidence-Based Practice

Quality Improvement

Safety

Informatics

Peer Review: _____   Faculty Review: _____

Grade Tracker

<table>
<tr><td></td><td></td><td></td><td></td><td></td><td></td><td></td><td></td><td></td><td></td><td></td><td></td><td></td><td></td><td></td><td></td></tr>
</table>

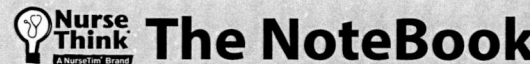

Related Concepts	**Related Exemplars/Diseases**

Reading/Resources - Clinical Judgment	**Class/Lab/Clinical – Clinical Judgment**

Priority Assessments or Cues	**Priority Labs & Diagnostics**	**Priority Nursing Interventions**
1	1	1
2	2	2
3	3	3

Priority Medications	**Priority Potential & Actual Complications**	**Priority Collaborative Goals**
1	1	1
2	2	2
3	3	3

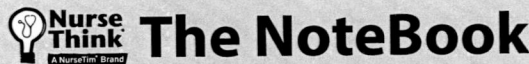
NurseThink® Quick

NEXT GEN LEARNING – NCLEX® TEST PLAN

Safe and Effective Care: Management of Care, Coordinated Care, Safety and Infection Control

Health Promotion and Maintenance

Psychosocial Integrity

Physiological Integrity: Basic Care and Comfort, Pharmacological and Parenteral Therapies, Reduction of Risk Potential, and Physiological Adaptation

QUALITY AND SAFETY COMPETENCIES

Patient-Centered Care

Teamwork and Collaboration

Evidence-Based Practice

Quality Improvement

Safety

Informatics

Peer Review: _____   Faculty Review: _____

Grade Tracker

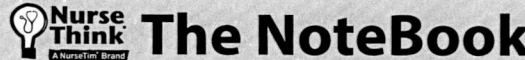 **The NoteBook** **Multiple Sclerosis**

Related Concepts	Related Exemplars/Diseases

Reading/Resources - Clinical Judgment	Class/Lab/Clinical – Clinical Judgment

Priority Assessments or Cues
1
2
3

Priority Labs & Diagnostics
1
2
3

Priority Nursing Interventions
1
2
3

Priority Medications
1
2
3

Priority Potential & Actual Complications
1
2
3

Priority Collaborative Goals
1
2
3

Copyright © 2021 by NurseTim, Inc. All rights reserved. No reproduction or distribution allowed.

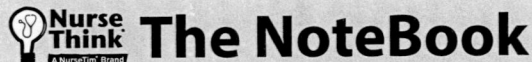
NurseThink® Quick

Multiple Sclerosis: Symptoms	**Multiple Sclerosis: Patho**	
Insular	MS attacks the Myelin Sheath, resulting in plaques.	
Intention tremor		
Nystagmus		
Slurred speech		
Uthoff's phenomenon		
Lhermitte's sign		
Ataxia		
Rebound		

NEXT GEN LEARNING – NCLEX® TEST PLAN

Safe and Effective Care: Management of Care, Coordinated Care, Safety and Infection Control

Health Promotion and Maintenance

Psychosocial Integrity

Physiological Integrity: Basic Care and Comfort, Pharmacological and Parenteral Therapies, Reduction of Risk Potential, and Physiological Adaptation

QUALITY AND SAFETY COMPETENCIES

Patient-Centered Care

Teamwork and Collaboration

Evidence-Based Practice

Quality Improvement

Safety

Informatics

Peer Review: _____   Faculty Review: _____

Grade Tracker

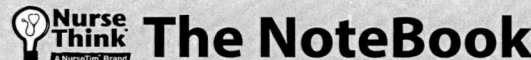
Related Concepts	Related Exemplars/Diseases

Reading/Resources - Clinical Judgment	Class/Lab/Clinical – Clinical Judgment

Priority Assessments or Cues

1

2

3

Priority Labs & Diagnostics

1

2

3

Priority Nursing Interventions

1

2

3

Priority Medications

1

2

3

Priority Potential & Actual Complications

1

2

3

Priority Collaborative Goals

1

2

3

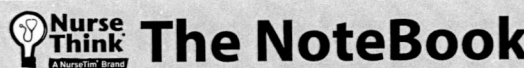
NurseThink® Quick

NEXT GEN LEARNING – NCLEX® TEST PLAN

Safe and Effective Care: Management of Care, Coordinated Care, Safety and Infection Control

Health Promotion and Maintenance

Psychosocial Integrity

Physiological Integrity: Basic Care and Comfort, Pharmacological and Parenteral Therapies, Reduction of Risk Potential, and Physiological Adaptation

QUALITY AND SAFETY COMPETENCIES

Patient-Centered Care

Teamwork and Collaboration

Evidence-Based Practice

Quality Improvement

Safety

Informatics

Peer Review: _____   Faculty Review: _____

Grade Tracker

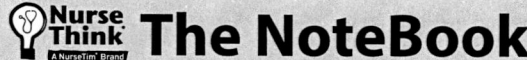

Related Concepts	Related Exemplars/Diseases

Reading/Resources - Clinical Judgment	Class/Lab/Clinical – Clinical Judgment
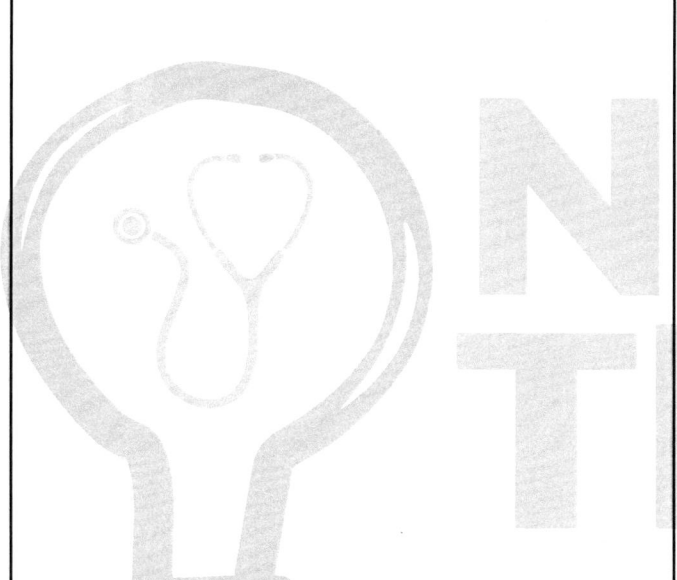	

Priority Assessments or Cues	Priority Labs & Diagnostics	Priority Nursing Interventions
1	1	1
2	2	2
3	3	3

Priority Medications	Priority Potential & Actual Complications	Priority Collaborative Goals
1	1	1
2	2	2
3	3	3

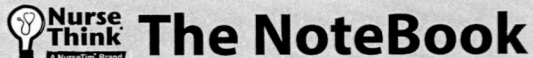
NurseThink® Quick

Parkinson's Medications	Parkinson's Symptoms	
Ali Loves Boxing Matches	*Parkinson's*	
Amantadine	**P**ill rolling	
Levodopa	**A**kinesis	
Bromocriptine	**R**igidity	
MAO inhibitors	**K**yphosis	
	Instability	
	Neck titubation	
	Shuffling gait	
	Oculogyric crisis	
	Nose tab (glabellar)	
	Small writing	

NEXT GEN LEARNING – NCLEX® TEST PLAN

Safe and Effective Care: Management of Care, Coordinated Care, Safety and Infection Control

Health Promotion and Maintenance

Psychosocial Integrity

Physiological Integrity: Basic Care and Comfort, Pharmacological and Parenteral Therapies, Reduction of Risk Potential, and Physiological Adaptation

QUALITY AND SAFETY COMPETENCIES

Patient-Centered Care

Teamwork and Collaboration

Evidence-Based Practice

Quality Improvement

Safety

Informatics

Peer Review: _____   Faculty Review: _____

Grade Tracker

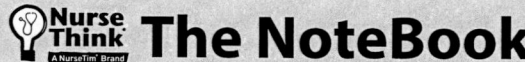
Related Concepts

Related Exemplars/Diseases

Reading/Resources - Clinical Judgment

Class/Lab/Clinical – Clinical Judgment

Priority Assessments or Cues

1

2

3

Priority Labs & Diagnostics

1

2

3

Priority Nursing Interventions

1

2

3

Priority Medications

1

2

3

Priority Potential & Actual Complications

1

2

3

Priority Collaborative Goals

1

2

3

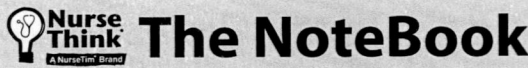
NurseThink® Quick

NEXT GEN LEARNING – NCLEX® TEST PLAN

Safe and Effective Care: Management of Care, Coordinated Care, Safety and Infection Control

Health Promotion and Maintenance

Psychosocial Integrity

Physiological Integrity: Basic Care and Comfort, Pharmacological and Parenteral Therapies, Reduction of Risk Potential, and Physiological Adaptation

QUALITY AND SAFETY COMPETENCIES

Patient-Centered Care

Teamwork and Collaboration

Evidence-Based Practice

Quality Improvement

Safety

Informatics

Peer Review: _____   Faculty Review: _____

Grade Tracker

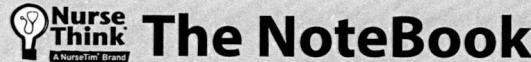
Related Concepts

Related Exemplars/Diseases

Reading/Resources - Clinical Judgment

Class/Lab/Clinical – Clinical Judgment

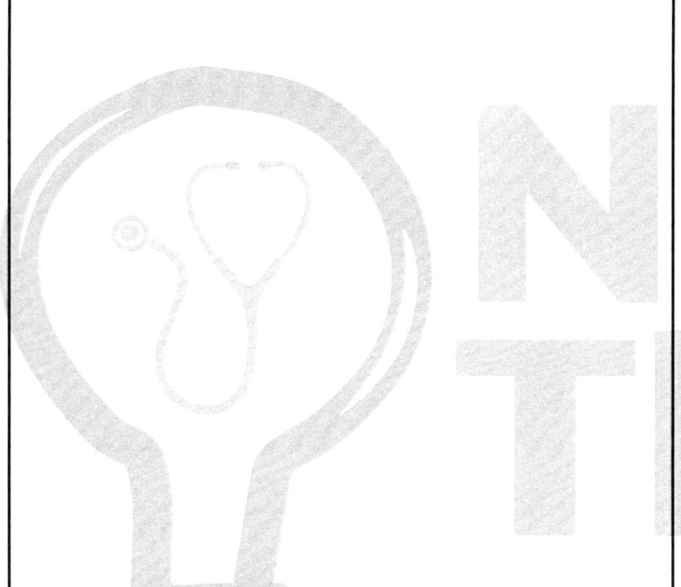

Priority Assessments or Cues
1
2
3

Priority Labs & Diagnostics
1
2
3

Priority Nursing Interventions
1
2
3

Priority Medications
1
2
3

Priority Potential & Actual Complications
1
2
3

Priority Collaborative Goals
1
2
3

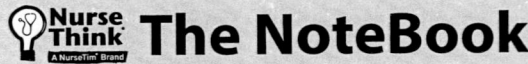
NurseThink® Quick

Seizure: Quick History Taking

Fact
Focus: generalized vs. local activity
Activity: tonic clonic vs. absence
Color: red, blue, ashen
Time: length of seizure

NEXT GEN LEARNING – NCLEX® TEST PLAN

Safe and Effective Care: Management of Care, Coordinated Care, Safety and Infection Control

Health Promotion and Maintenance

Psychosocial Integrity

Physiological Integrity: Basic Care and Comfort, Pharmacological and Parenteral Therapies, Reduction of Risk Potential, and Physiological Adaptation

QUALITY AND SAFETY COMPETENCIES

Patient-Centered Care

Teamwork and Collaboration

Evidence-Based Practice

Quality Improvement

Safety

Informatics

Peer Review: _____   Faculty Review: _____

Grade Tracker

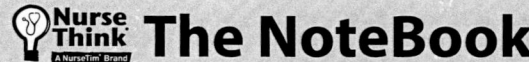

Related Concepts

Related Exemplars/Diseases

Reading/Resources - Clinical Judgment

Class/Lab/Clinical – Clinical Judgment

Priority Assessments or Cues

1

2

3

Priority Labs & Diagnostics

1

2

3

Priority Nursing Interventions

1

2

3

Priority Medications

1

2

3

Priority Potential & Actual Complications

1

2

3

Priority Collaborative Goals

1

2

3

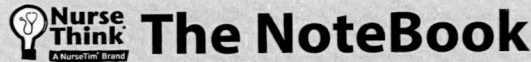

NurseThink® Quick

NEXT GEN LEARNING – NCLEX® TEST PLAN

Safe and Effective Care: Management of Care, Coordinated Care, Safety and Infection Control

Health Promotion and Maintenance

Psychosocial Integrity

Physiological Integrity: Basic Care and Comfort, Pharmacological and Parenteral Therapies, Reduction of Risk Potential, and Physiological Adaptation

QUALITY AND SAFETY COMPETENCIES

Patient-Centered Care

Teamwork and Collaboration

Evidence-Based Practice

Quality Improvement

Safety

Informatics

Peer Review: _____   Faculty Review: _____

Grade Tracker

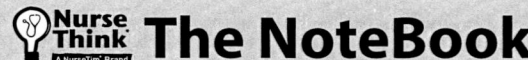

Related Concepts	Related Exemplars/Diseases

Reading/Resources - Clinical Judgment	Class/Lab/Clinical – Clinical Judgment

Priority Assessments or Cues

1

2

3

Priority Labs & Diagnostics

1

2

3

Priority Nursing Interventions

1

2

3

Priority Medications

1

2

3

Priority Potential & Actual Complications

1

2

3

Priority Collaborative Goals

1

2

3

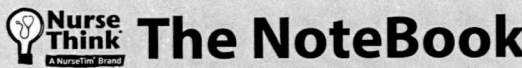
NurseThink® Quick

NEXT GEN LEARNING – NCLEX® TEST PLAN

Safe and Effective Care: Management of Care, Coordinated Care, Safety and Infection Control

Health Promotion and Maintenance

Psychosocial Integrity

Physiological Integrity: Basic Care and Comfort, Pharmacological and Parenteral Therapies, Reduction of Risk Potential, and Physiological Adaptation

QUALITY AND SAFETY COMPETENCIES

Patient-Centered Care

Teamwork and Collaboration

Evidence-Based Practice

Quality Improvement

Safety

Informatics

Peer Review: _____   Faculty Review: _____

Grade Tracker

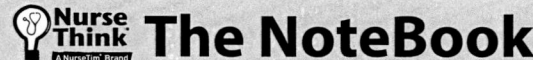

Related Concepts	Related Exemplars/Diseases

Reading/Resources - Clinical Judgment	Class/Lab/Clinical – Clinical Judgment

Priority Assessments or Cues	Priority Labs & Diagnostics	Priority Nursing Interventions
1	1	1
2	2	2
3	3	3

Priority Medications	Priority Potential & Actual Complications	Priority Collaborative Goals
1	1	1
2	2	2
3	3	3

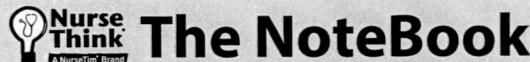
NurseThink® Quick

Cataracts: Differential		
CATARAct		
Congenital		
Aging		
Toxicity (Steroids, etc.)		
Accidents		
Radiation		
Abnormal metabolism		

NEXT GEN LEARNING – NCLEX® TEST PLAN

Safe and Effective Care: Management of Care, Coordinated Care, Safety and Infection Control

Health Promotion and Maintenance

Psychosocial Integrity

Physiological Integrity: Basic Care and Comfort, Pharmacological and Parenteral Therapies, Reduction of Risk Potential, and Physiological Adaptation

QUALITY AND SAFETY COMPETENCIES

Patient-Centered Care

Teamwork and Collaboration

Evidence-Based Practice

Quality Improvement

Safety

Informatics

Peer Review: _____   Faculty Review: _____

Grade Tracker

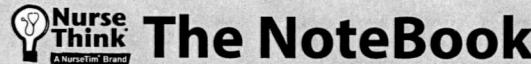

Related Concepts	Related Exemplars/Diseases

Reading/Resources - Clinical Judgment	Class/Lab/Clinical – Clinical Judgment

Priority Assessments or Cues	Priority Labs & Diagnostics	Priority Nursing Interventions
1	1	1
2	2	2
3	3	3

Priority Medications	Priority Potential & Actual Complications	Priority Collaborative Goals
1	1	1
2	2	2
3	3	3

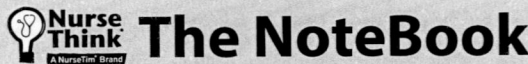
NurseThink® Quick

NEXT GEN LEARNING – NCLEX® TEST PLAN

Safe and Effective Care: Management of Care, Coordinated Care, Safety and Infection Control

Health Promotion and Maintenance

Psychosocial Integrity

Physiological Integrity: Basic Care and Comfort, Pharmacological and Parenteral Therapies, Reduction of Risk Potential, and Physiological Adaptation

QUALITY AND SAFETY COMPETENCIES

Patient-Centered Care

Teamwork and Collaboration

Evidence-Based Practice

Quality Improvement

Safety

Informatics

Peer Review: _____ Faculty Review: _____

Grade Tracker

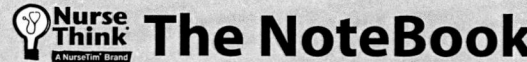
Related Concepts	Related Exemplars/Diseases

Reading/Resources - Clinical Judgment	Class/Lab/Clinical – Clinical Judgment

Priority Assessments or Cues	Priority Labs & Diagnostics	Priority Nursing Interventions
1	1	1
2	2	2
3	3	3

Priority Medications	Priority Potential & Actual Complications	Priority Collaborative Goals
1	1	1
2	2	2
3	3	3

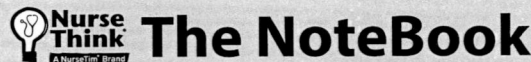 **The NoteBook**

Glaucoma

NurseThink® Quick

NEXT GEN LEARNING – NCLEX® TEST PLAN

Safe and Effective Care: Management of Care, Coordinated Care, Safety and Infection Control

Health Promotion and Maintenance

Psychosocial Integrity

Physiological Integrity: Basic Care and Comfort, Pharmacological and Parenteral Therapies, Reduction of Risk Potential, and Physiological Adaptation

QUALITY AND SAFETY COMPETENCIES

Patient-Centered Care

Teamwork and Collaboration

Evidence-Based Practice

Quality Improvement

Safety

Informatics

Peer Review: _____   Faculty Review: _____

Grade Tracker

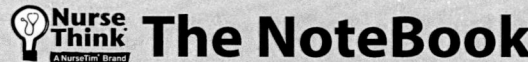

Related Concepts	Related Exemplars/Diseases

Reading/Resources - Clinical Judgment	Class/Lab/Clinical – Clinical Judgment

Priority Assessments or Cues	Priority Labs & Diagnostics	Priority Nursing Interventions
1	1	1
2	2	2
3	3	3

Priority Medications	Priority Potential & Actual Complications	Priority Collaborative Goals
1	1	1
2	2	2
3	3	3

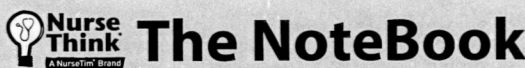
NurseThink® Quick

NEXT GEN LEARNING – NCLEX® TEST PLAN

Safe and Effective Care: Management of Care, Coordinated Care, Safety and Infection Control

Health Promotion and Maintenance

Psychosocial Integrity

Physiological Integrity: Basic Care and Comfort, Pharmacological and Parenteral Therapies, Reduction of Risk Potential, and Physiological Adaptation

QUALITY AND SAFETY COMPETENCIES

Patient-Centered Care

Teamwork and Collaboration

Evidence-Based Practice

Quality Improvement

Safety

Informatics

Peer Review: _____   Faculty Review: _____

Grade Tracker

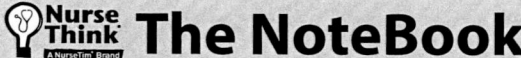
Related Concepts

Related Exemplars/Diseases

Reading/Resources - Clinical Judgment

Class/Lab/Clinical – Clinical Judgment

Priority Assessments or Cues

1

2

3

Priority Labs & Diagnostics

1

2

3

Priority Nursing Interventions

1

2

3

Priority Medications

1

2

3

Priority Potential & Actual Complications

1

2

3

Priority Collaborative Goals

1

2

3

NurseThink® Quick

NEXT GEN LEARNING – NCLEX® TEST PLAN

Safe and Effective Care: Management of Care, Coordinated Care, Safety and Infection Control

Health Promotion and Maintenance

Psychosocial Integrity

Physiological Integrity: Basic Care and Comfort, Pharmacological and Parenteral Therapies, Reduction of Risk Potential, and Physiological Adaptation

QUALITY AND SAFETY COMPETENCIES

Patient-Centered Care

Teamwork and Collaboration

Evidence-Based Practice

Quality Improvement

Safety

Informatics

Peer Review: _____   Faculty Review: _____

Grade Tracker

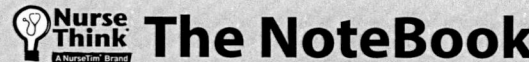
Related Concepts

Related Exemplars/Diseases

Reading/Resources - Clinical Judgment

Class/Lab/Clinical – Clinical Judgment

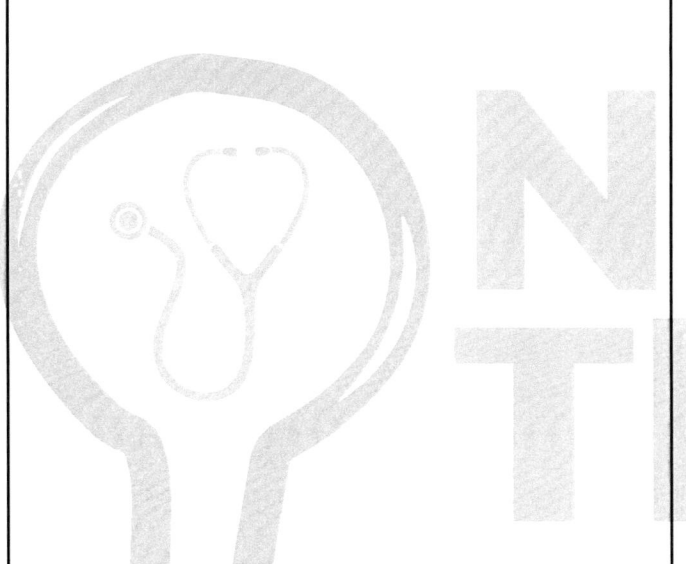

Priority Assessments or Cues	Priority Labs & Diagnostics	Priority Nursing Interventions
1	1	1
2	2	2
3	3	3

Priority Medications	Priority Potential & Actual Complications	Priority Collaborative Goals
1	1	1
2	2	2
3	3	3

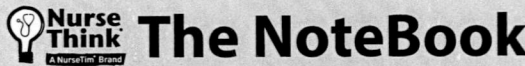
NurseThink® Quick

NEXT GEN LEARNING – NCLEX® TEST PLAN

Safe and Effective Care: Management of Care, Coordinated Care, Safety and Infection Control

Health Promotion and Maintenance

Psychosocial Integrity

Physiological Integrity: Basic Care and Comfort, Pharmacological and Parenteral Therapies, Reduction of Risk Potential, and Physiological Adaptation

QUALITY AND SAFETY COMPETENCIES

Patient-Centered Care

Teamwork and Collaboration

Evidence-Based Practice

Quality Improvement

Safety

Informatics

Peer Review: _____   Faculty Review: _____

Grade Tracker

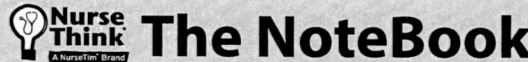
Related Concepts	Related Exemplars/Diseases

Reading/Resources - Clinical Judgment	Class/Lab/Clinical – Clinical Judgment

Priority Assessments or Cues
1
2
3

Priority Labs & Diagnostics
1
2
3

Priority Nursing Interventions
1
2
3

Priority Medications
1
2
3

Priority Potential & Actual Complications
1
2
3

Priority Collaborative Goals
1
2
3

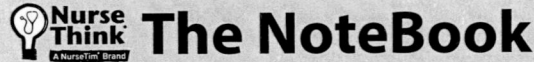
NurseThink® Quick

<table>
<tr><td></td><td></td><td></td></tr>
</table>

NEXT GEN LEARNING – NCLEX® TEST PLAN

Safe and Effective Care: Management of Care, Coordinated Care, Safety and Infection Control

Health Promotion and Maintenance

Psychosocial Integrity

Physiological Integrity: Basic Care and Comfort, Pharmacological and Parenteral Therapies, Reduction of Risk Potential, and Physiological Adaptation

QUALITY AND SAFETY COMPETENCIES

Patient-Centered Care

Teamwork and Collaboration

Evidence-Based Practice

Quality Improvement

Safety

Informatics

Peer Review: _____   Faculty Review: _____

Grade Tracker

<table>
<tr><td></td><td></td><td></td><td></td><td></td><td></td><td></td><td></td><td></td><td></td><td></td><td></td><td></td><td></td><td></td></tr>
</table>

Related Concepts

Related Exemplars/Diseases

Reading/Resources - Clinical Judgment

Class/Lab/Clinical – Clinical Judgment

Priority Assessments or Cues

1

2

3

Priority Labs & Diagnostics

1

2

3

Priority Nursing Interventions

1

2

3

Priority Medications

1

2

3

Priority Potential & Actual Complications

1

2

3

Priority Collaborative Goals

1

2

3

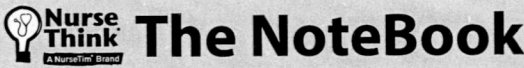
NurseThink® Quick

NEXT GEN LEARNING – NCLEX® TEST PLAN

Safe and Effective Care: Management of Care, Coordinated Care, Safety and Infection Control

Health Promotion and Maintenance

Psychosocial Integrity

Physiological Integrity: Basic Care and Comfort, Pharmacological and Parenteral Therapies, Reduction of Risk Potential, and Physiological Adaptation

QUALITY AND SAFETY COMPETENCIES

Patient-Centered Care

Teamwork and Collaboration

Evidence-Based Practice

Quality Improvement

Safety

Informatics

Peer Review: _____   Faculty Review: _____

Grade Tracker

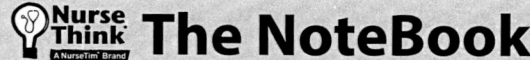
Related Concepts	Related Exemplars/Diseases

Reading/Resources - Clinical Judgment	Class/Lab/Clinical – Clinical Judgment

Priority Assessments or Cues	Priority Labs & Diagnostics	Priority Nursing Interventions
1	1	1
2	2	2
3	3	3

Priority Medications	Priority Potential & Actual Complications	Priority Collaborative Goals
1	1	1
2	2	2
3	3	3

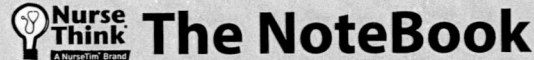
NurseThink® Quick

Appendicitis: Assessment
Pains
Pain, RLQ
Anorexia
Increased temperature
Nausea
Signs (McBurney's Psoas)

NEXT GEN LEARNING – NCLEX® TEST PLAN

Safe and Effective Care: Management of Care, Coordinated Care, Safety and Infection Control

Health Promotion and Maintenance

Psychosocial Integrity

Physiological Integrity: Basic Care and Comfort, Pharmacological and Parenteral Therapies, Reduction of Risk Potential, and Physiological Adaptation

QUALITY AND SAFETY COMPETENCIES

Patient-Centered Care

Teamwork and Collaboration

Evidence-Based Practice

Quality Improvement

Safety

Informatics

Peer Review: _____   Faculty Review: _____

Grade Tracker

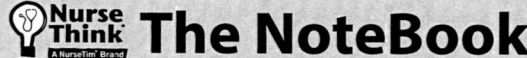
Related Concepts	Related Exemplars/Diseases

Reading/Resources - Clinical Judgment	Class/Lab/Clinical – Clinical Judgment
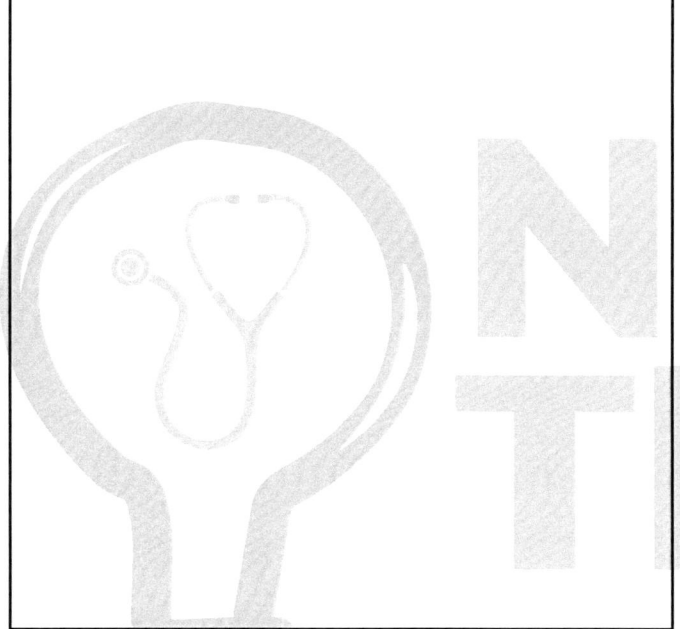	

Priority Assessments or Cues	Priority Labs & Diagnostics	Priority Nursing Interventions
1	1	1
2	2	2
3	3	3

Priority Medications	Priority Potential & Actual Complications	Priority Collaborative Goals
1	1	1
2	2	2
3	3	3

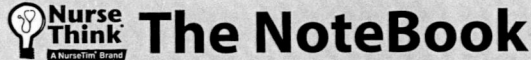
NurseThink® Quick

Cholelithiasis: Risk Factors	**Charcot's Triad (gallstones)**	
5 F's **F**emale **F**air skinned **F**at **F**orty **F**ertile	**3 C's** **C**olor change (jaundice) **C**olic (biliary) pain **C**hills and fever	

NEXT GEN LEARNING – NCLEX® TEST PLAN

Safe and Effective Care: Management of Care, Coordinated Care, Safety and Infection Control

Health Promotion and Maintenance

Psychosocial Integrity

Physiological Integrity: Basic Care and Comfort, Pharmacological and Parenteral Therapies, Reduction of Risk Potential, and Physiological Adaptation

QUALITY AND SAFETY COMPETENCIES

Patient-Centered Care

Teamwork and Collaboration

Evidence-Based Practice

Quality Improvement

Safety

Informatics

Peer Review: _____   Faculty Review: _____

Grade Tracker

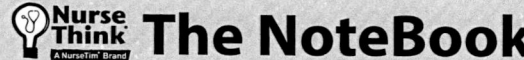
Related Concepts	**Related Exemplars/Diseases**

Reading/Resources - Clinical Judgment	**Class/Lab/Clinical – Clinical Judgment**

Priority Assessments or Cues

1

2

3

Priority Labs & Diagnostics

1

2

3

Priority Nursing Interventions

1

2

3

Priority Medications

1

2

3

Priority Potential & Actual Complications

1

2

3

Priority Collaborative Goals

1

2

3

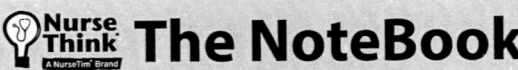
NurseThink® Quick

NEXT GEN LEARNING – NCLEX® TEST PLAN

Safe and Effective Care: Management of Care, Coordinated Care, Safety and Infection Control

Health Promotion and Maintenance

Psychosocial Integrity

Physiological Integrity: Basic Care and Comfort, Pharmacological and Parenteral Therapies, Reduction of Risk Potential, and Physiological Adaptation

QUALITY AND SAFETY COMPETENCIES

Patient-Centered Care

Teamwork and Collaboration

Evidence-Based Practice

Quality Improvement

Safety

Informatics

Peer Review: _____   Faculty Review: _____

Grade Tracker

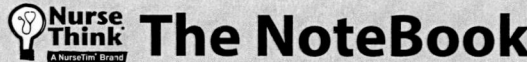

Related Concepts	Related Exemplars/Diseases

Reading/Resources - Clinical Judgment	Class/Lab/Clinical – Clinical Judgment
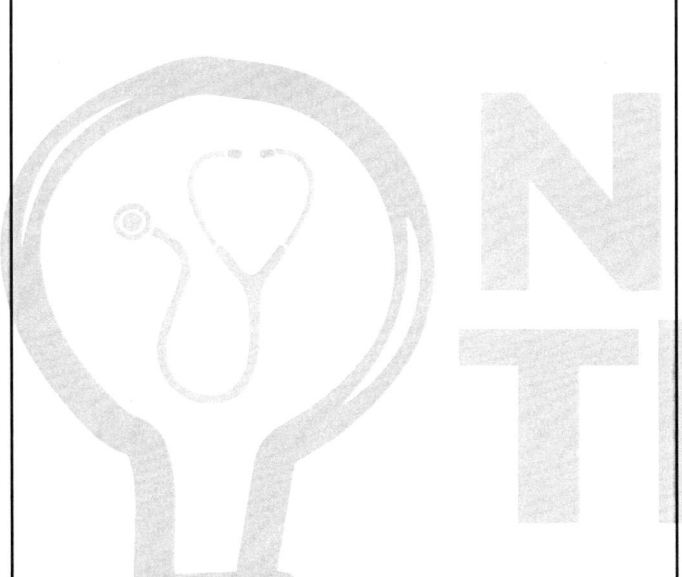	

Priority Assessments or Cues	Priority Labs & Diagnostics	Priority Nursing Interventions
1	1	1
2	2	2
3	3	3

Priority Medications	Priority Potential & Actual Complications	Priority Collaborative Goals
1	1	1
2	2	2
3	3	3

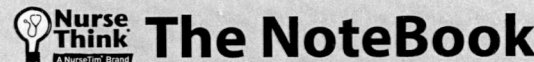
NurseThink® Quick

NEXT GEN LEARNING – NCLEX® TEST PLAN

Safe and Effective Care: Management of Care, Coordinated Care, Safety and Infection Control

Health Promotion and Maintenance

Psychosocial Integrity

Physiological Integrity: Basic Care and Comfort, Pharmacological and Parenteral Therapies, Reduction of Risk Potential, and Physiological Adaptation

QUALITY AND SAFETY COMPETENCIES

Patient-Centered Care

Teamwork and Collaboration

Evidence-Based Practice

Quality Improvement

Safety

Informatics

Peer Review: _____   Faculty Review: _____

Grade Tracker

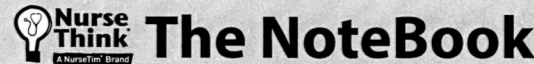
Related Concepts	**Related Exemplars/Diseases**

Reading/Resources - Clinical Judgment	**Class/Lab/Clinical – Clinical Judgment**

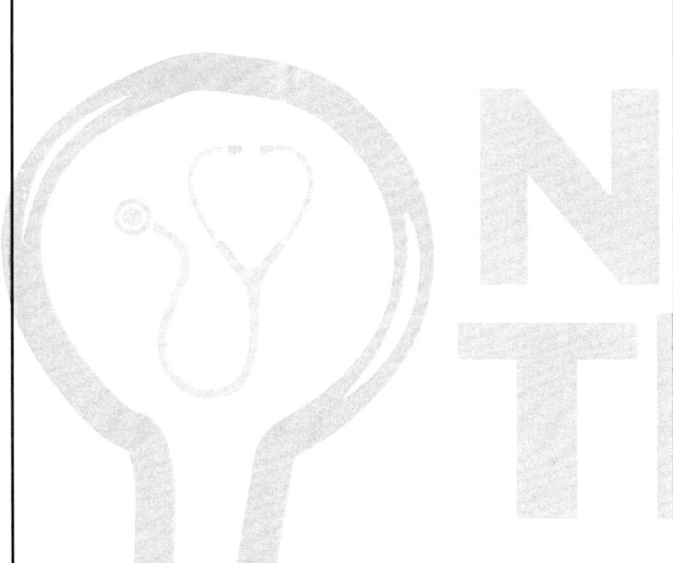

Priority Assessments or Cues	**Priority Labs & Diagnostics**	**Priority Nursing Interventions**
1	1	1
2	2	2
3	3	3

Priority Medications	**Priority Potential & Actual Complications**	**Priority Collaborative Goals**
1	1	1
2	2	2
3	3	3

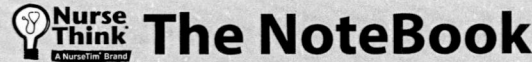
NurseThink® Quick

NEXT GEN LEARNING – NCLEX® TEST PLAN

Safe and Effective Care: Management of Care, Coordinated Care, Safety and Infection Control

Health Promotion and Maintenance

Psychosocial Integrity

Physiological Integrity: Basic Care and Comfort, Pharmacological and Parenteral Therapies, Reduction of Risk Potential, and Physiological Adaptation

---

QUALITY AND SAFETY COMPETENCIES

Patient-Centered Care

Teamwork and Collaboration

Evidence-Based Practice

Quality Improvement

Safety

Informatics

Peer Review: _____   Faculty Review: _____

Grade Tracker

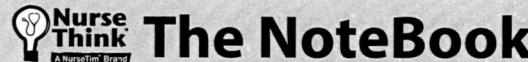
Related Concepts	Related Exemplars/Diseases

Reading/Resources - Clinical Judgment	Class/Lab/Clinical – Clinical Judgment

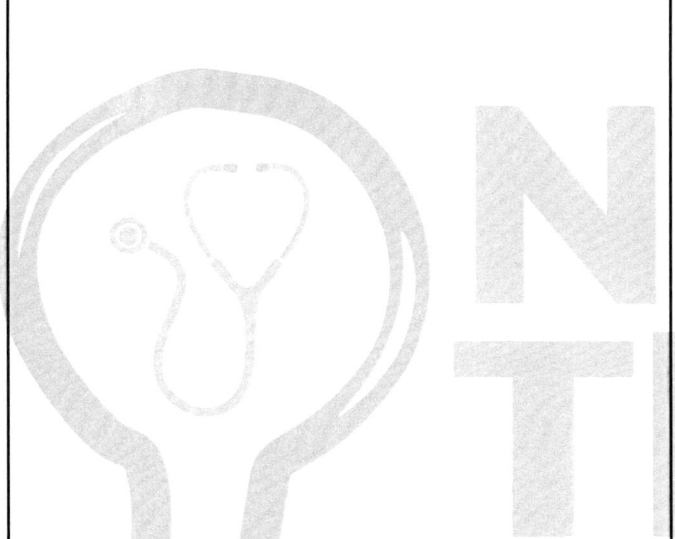

Priority Assessments or Cues	Priority Labs & Diagnostics	Priority Nursing Interventions
1	1	1
2	2	2
3	3	3

Priority Medications	Priority Potential & Actual Complications	Priority Collaborative Goals
1	1	1
2	2	2
3	3	3

NurseThink® Quick

NEXT GEN LEARNING – NCLEX® TEST PLAN

Safe and Effective Care: Management of Care, Coordinated Care, Safety and Infection Control

Health Promotion and Maintenance

Psychosocial Integrity

Physiological Integrity: Basic Care and Comfort, Pharmacological and Parenteral Therapies, Reduction of Risk Potential, and Physiological Adaptation

QUALITY AND SAFETY COMPETENCIES

Patient-Centered Care

Teamwork and Collaboration

Evidence-Based Practice

Quality Improvement

Safety

Informatics

Peer Review: _____   Faculty Review: _____

Grade Tracker

Related Concepts

Related Exemplars/Diseases

Reading/Resources - Clinical Judgment

Class/Lab/Clinical – Clinical Judgment

Priority Assessments or Cues

1

2

3

Priority Labs & Diagnostics

1

2

3

Priority Nursing Interventions

1

2

3

Priority Medications

1

2

3

Priority Potential & Actual Complications

1

2

3

Priority Collaborative Goals

1

2

3

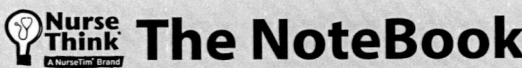
NurseThink® Quick

NEXT GEN LEARNING – NCLEX® TEST PLAN

Safe and Effective Care: Management of Care, Coordinated Care, Safety and Infection Control

Health Promotion and Maintenance

Psychosocial Integrity

Physiological Integrity: Basic Care and Comfort, Pharmacological and Parenteral Therapies, Reduction of Risk Potential, and Physiological Adaptation

QUALITY AND SAFETY COMPETENCIES

Patient-Centered Care

Teamwork and Collaboration

Evidence-Based Practice

Quality Improvement

Safety

Informatics

Peer Review: _____   Faculty Review: _____

Grade Tracker

Related Concepts	Related Exemplars/Diseases

Reading/Resources - Clinical Judgment	Class/Lab/Clinical – Clinical Judgment
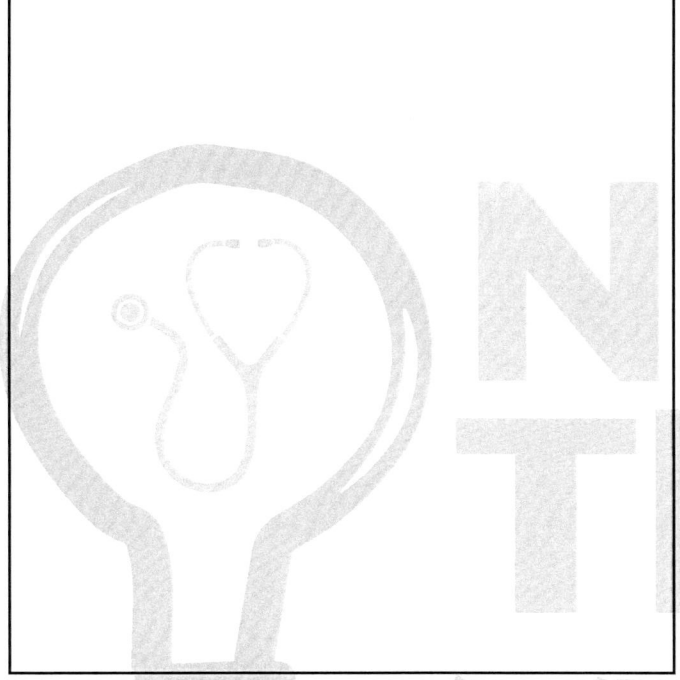	

Priority Assessments or Cues

1

2

3

Priority Labs & Diagnostics

1

2

3

Priority Nursing Interventions

1

2

3

Priority Medications

1

2

3

Priority Potential & Actual Complications

1

2

3

Priority Collaborative Goals

1

2

3

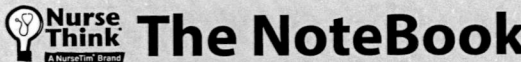
NurseThink® Quick

<table>
<tr><td></td><td></td><td></td></tr>
</table>

NEXT GEN LEARNING – NCLEX® TEST PLAN

Safe and Effective Care: Management of Care, Coordinated Care, Safety and Infection Control

Health Promotion and Maintenance

Psychosocial Integrity

Physiological Integrity: Basic Care and Comfort, Pharmacological and Parenteral Therapies, Reduction of Risk Potential, and Physiological Adaptation

QUALITY AND SAFETY COMPETENCIES

Patient-Centered Care

Teamwork and Collaboration

Evidence-Based Practice

Quality Improvement

Safety

Informatics

Peer Review: _____   Faculty Review: _____

Grade Tracker

<table>
<tr><td></td><td></td><td></td><td></td><td></td><td></td><td></td><td></td><td></td><td></td><td></td><td></td><td></td><td></td><td></td><td></td></tr>
</table>

Related Concepts

Related Exemplars/Diseases

Reading/Resources - Clinical Judgment

Class/Lab/Clinical – Clinical Judgment

Priority Assessments or Cues

1

2

3

Priority Labs & Diagnostics

1

2

3

Priority Nursing Interventions

1

2

3

Priority Medications

1

2

3

Priority Potential & Actual Complications

1

2

3

Priority Collaborative Goals

1

2

3

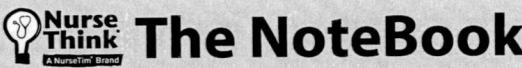
NurseThink® Quick

NEXT GEN LEARNING – NCLEX® TEST PLAN

Safe and Effective Care: Management of Care, Coordinated Care, Safety and Infection Control

Health Promotion and Maintenance

Psychosocial Integrity

Physiological Integrity: Basic Care and Comfort, Pharmacological and Parenteral Therapies, Reduction of Risk Potential, and Physiological Adaptation

QUALITY AND SAFETY COMPETENCIES

Patient-Centered Care

Teamwork and Collaboration

Evidence-Based Practice

Quality Improvement

Safety

Informatics

Peer Review: _____   Faculty Review: _____

Grade Tracker

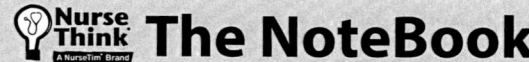
Related Concepts	Related Exemplars/Diseases

Reading/Resources - Clinical Judgment	Class/Lab/Clinical – Clinical Judgment

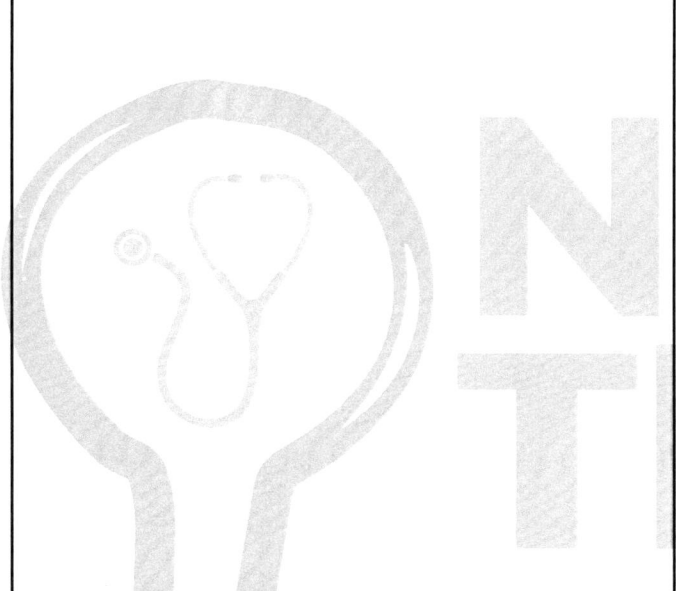

Priority Assessments or Cues	Priority Labs & Diagnostics	Priority Nursing Interventions
1	1	1
2	2	2
3	3	3

Priority Medications	Priority Potential & Actual Complications	Priority Collaborative Goals
1	1	1
2	2	2
3	3	3

NurseThink® Quick

Immunization Reaction: Signs and Symptoms		
Fisher Flag		
Fever		
Itching		
Stiffness		
Headache		
Edema		
Redness		
Fussy		
Localized tenderness		
Appetite decrease		
General aches and pains		

NEXT GEN LEARNING – NCLEX® TEST PLAN

Safe and Effective Care: Management of Care, Coordinated Care, Safety and Infection Control

Health Promotion and Maintenance

Psychosocial Integrity

Physiological Integrity: Basic Care and Comfort, Pharmacological and Parenteral Therapies, Reduction of Risk Potential, and Physiological Adaptation

QUALITY AND SAFETY COMPETENCIES

Patient-Centered Care

Teamwork and Collaboration

Evidence-Based Practice

Quality Improvement

Safety

Informatics

Peer Review: _____   Faculty Review: _____

Grade Tracker

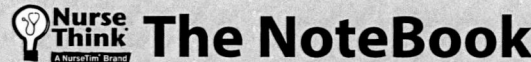
Related Concepts

Related Exemplars/Diseases

Reading/Resources - Clinical Judgment

Class/Lab/Clinical – Clinical Judgment

Priority Assessments or Cues
1
2
3

Priority Labs & Diagnostics
1
2
3

Priority Nursing Interventions
1
2
3

Priority Medications
1
2
3

Priority Potential & Actual Complications
1
2
3

Priority Collaborative Goals
1
2
3

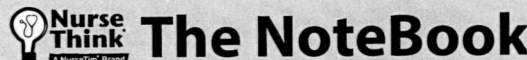
NurseThink® Quick

NEXT GEN LEARNING – NCLEX® TEST PLAN

Safe and Effective Care: Management of Care, Coordinated Care, Safety and Infection Control

Health Promotion and Maintenance

Psychosocial Integrity

Physiological Integrity: Basic Care and Comfort, Pharmacological and Parenteral Therapies, Reduction of Risk Potential, and Physiological Adaptation

QUALITY AND SAFETY COMPETENCIES

Patient-Centered Care

Teamwork and Collaboration

Evidence-Based Practice

Quality Improvement

Safety

Informatics

Peer Review: _____   Faculty Review: _____

Grade Tracker

Related Concepts

Related Exemplars/Diseases

Reading/Resources - Clinical Judgment

Class/Lab/Clinical – Clinical Judgment

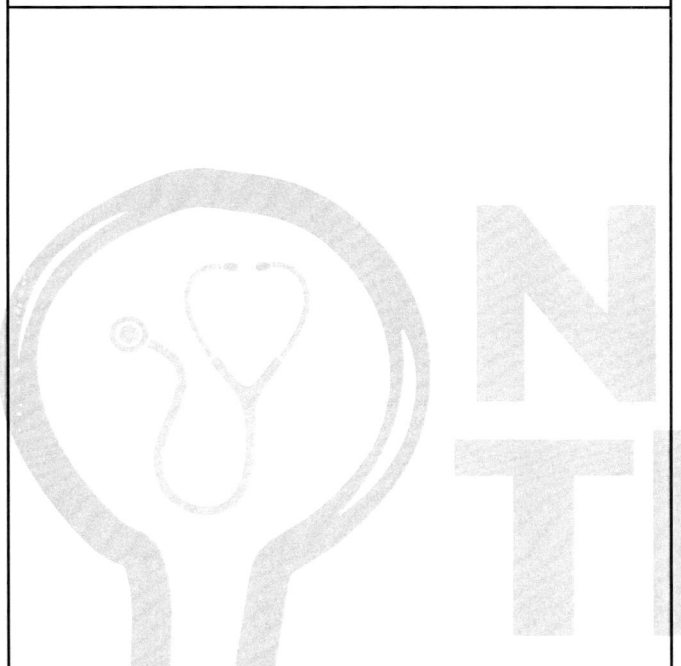

Priority Assessments or Cues

1

2

3

Priority Labs & Diagnostics

1

2

3

Priority Nursing Interventions

1

2

3

Priority Medications

1

2

3

Priority Potential & Actual Complications

1

2

3

Priority Collaborative Goals

1

2

3

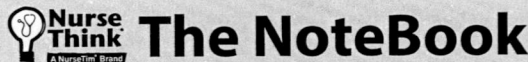
NurseThink® Quick

AIDS Pathogens	HIV Infection: High-Risk Groups	AIDS Dementia Complex
The Major Pathogens Concerning Complete T-Cell Collapse	***HHIV***	***AIDS***
Toxoplasma gondii	**H**omosexuals	**A**trophy of cortex
M. avium intracellular	**H**emophiliacs	**I**nfection/Inflammation
Pneumocystis carinii	**IV** drug abuses	**D**emyelination
Candida albicans		**S**ix months death
Cryptococcus neoformans		
Tuberculosis		
CMV		
Cryptosporidium parvum		

NEXT GEN LEARNING – NCLEX® TEST PLAN

Safe and Effective Care: Management of Care, Coordinated Care, Safety and Infection Control

Health Promotion and Maintenance

Psychosocial Integrity

Physiological Integrity: Basic Care and Comfort, Pharmacological and Parenteral Therapies, Reduction of Risk Potential, and Physiological Adaptation

QUALITY AND SAFETY COMPETENCIES

Patient-Centered Care

Teamwork and Collaboration

Evidence-Based Practice

Quality Improvement

Safety

Informatics

Peer Review: _____   Faculty Review: _____

Grade Tracker

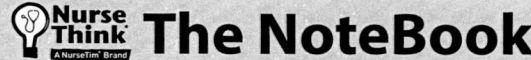

Related Concepts

Related Exemplars/Diseases

Reading/Resources - Clinical Judgment

Class/Lab/Clinical – Clinical Judgment

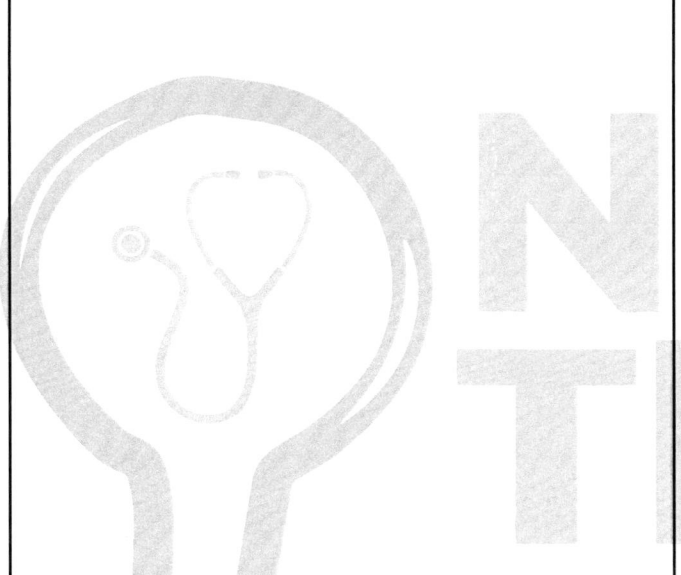

Priority Assessments or Cues
1

2

3

Priority Labs & Diagnostics
1

2

3

Priority Nursing Interventions
1

2

3

Priority Medications
1

2

3

Priority Potential & Actual Complications
1

2

3

Priority Collaborative Goals
1

2

3

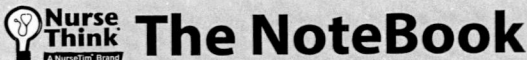
NurseThink® Quick

SLE: Symptoms	Lupus: Drug Inducing It	SLE: Factors Activating SLE
Soap Brain MD	***Hip***	***UV Prism***
Serositis	**H**ydralazine	**UV** (sunshine)
Oral ulcers	**I**NH	**P**regnancy
Arthritis	**P**rocainamide	**R**educed drug (steroid)
Photosensitivity		**I**nfection
Blood disorder		**S**tress
Renal disorder		**M**ore drugs
Antinuclear antibody test positive		
Immunologic disorder		
Neurologic disorder		
Malar rash		
Discoid rash		

NEXT GEN LEARNING – NCLEX® TEST PLAN

Safe and Effective Care: Management of Care, Coordinated Care, Safety and Infection Control

Health Promotion and Maintenance

Psychosocial Integrity

Physiological Integrity: Basic Care and Comfort, Pharmacological and Parenteral Therapies, Reduction of Risk Potential, and Physiological Adaptation

QUALITY AND SAFETY COMPETENCIES

Patient-Centered Care

Teamwork and Collaboration

Evidence-Based Practice

Quality Improvement

Safety

Informatics

Peer Review: _____   Faculty Review: _____

Grade Tracker

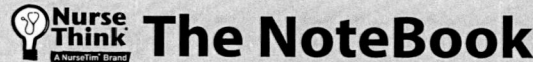
Related Concepts	Related Exemplars/Diseases

Reading/Resources - Clinical Judgment	Class/Lab/Clinical – Clinical Judgment

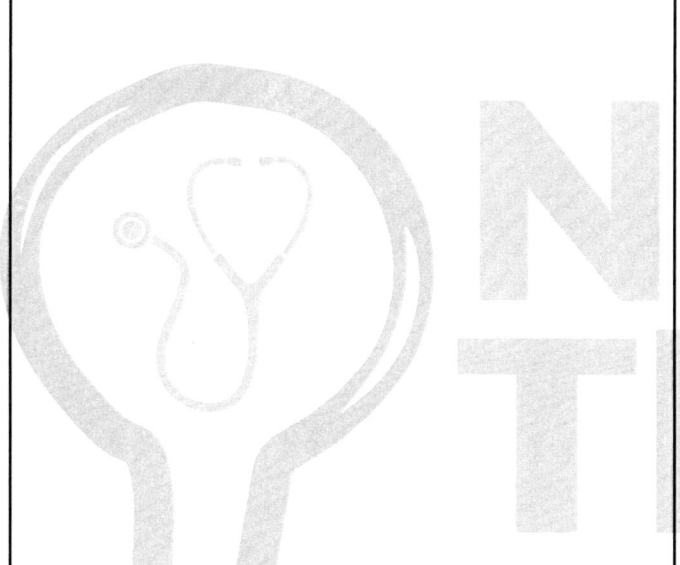

Priority Assessments or Cues

1

2

3

Priority Labs & Diagnostics

1

2

3

Priority Nursing Interventions

1

2

3

Priority Medications

1

2

3

Priority Potential & Actual Complications

1

2

3

Priority Collaborative Goals

1

2

3

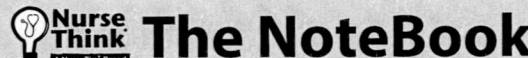

NurseThink® Quick

Rheumatoid Arthritis: Features

Rheumatoid

Ragocytes/Rheumatoid factor
HLA-DR4/Hla-Dw4
ESR increase/Extra-articular features
Ulnar deviation
Morning stiffness
Ankylosis/Atlantoaxial joint subluxation/
  Autoimmune/ANA
T-cells (CD4)/
Osteopenia
Inflammatory synovial tissue
Deformities

NEXT GEN LEARNING – NCLEX® TEST PLAN

Safe and Effective Care: Management of Care, Coordinated Care, Safety and Infection Control

Health Promotion and Maintenance

Psychosocial Integrity

Physiological Integrity: Basic Care and Comfort, Pharmacological and Parenteral Therapies, Reduction of Risk Potential, and Physiological Adaptation

QUALITY AND SAFETY COMPETENCIES

Patient-Centered Care

Teamwork and Collaboration

Evidence-Based Practice

Quality Improvement

Safety

Informatics

Peer Review: _____   Faculty Review: _____

Grade Tracker

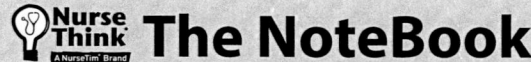
Related Concepts	Related Exemplars/Diseases

Reading/Resources - Clinical Judgment	Class/Lab/Clinical – Clinical Judgment
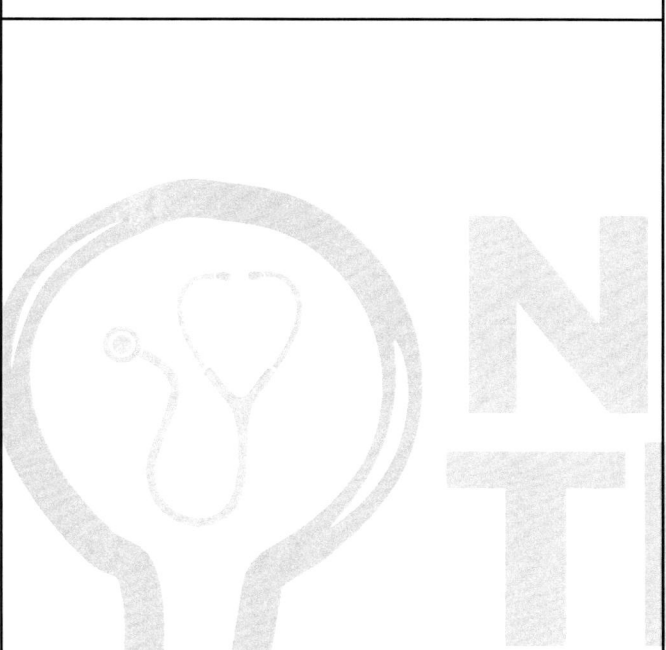	

Priority Assessments or Cues	Priority Labs & Diagnostics	Priority Nursing Interventions
1	1	1
2	2	2
3	3	3

Priority Medications	Priority Potential & Actual Complications	Priority Collaborative Goals
1	1	1
2	2	2
3	3	3

NurseThink® Quick

NEXT GEN LEARNING – NCLEX® TEST PLAN

Safe and Effective Care: Management of Care, Coordinated Care, Safety and Infection Control

Health Promotion and Maintenance

Psychosocial Integrity

Physiological Integrity: Basic Care and Comfort, Pharmacological and Parenteral Therapies, Reduction of Risk Potential, and Physiological Adaptation

QUALITY AND SAFETY COMPETENCIES

Patient-Centered Care

Teamwork and Collaboration

Evidence-Based Practice

Quality Improvement

Safety

Informatics

Peer Review: _____   Faculty Review: _____

Grade Tracker

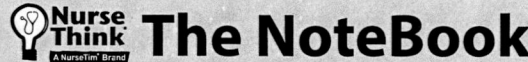
Related Concepts

Related Exemplars/Diseases

Reading/Resources - Clinical Judgment

Class/Lab/Clinical – Clinical Judgment

Priority Assessments or Cues

1

2

3

Priority Labs & Diagnostics

1

2

3

Priority Nursing Interventions

1

2

3

Priority Medications

1

2

3

Priority Potential & Actual Complications

1

2

3

Priority Collaborative Goals

1

2

3

NurseThink® Quick

NEXT GEN LEARNING – NCLEX® TEST PLAN

Safe and Effective Care: Management of Care, Coordinated Care, Safety and Infection Control

Health Promotion and Maintenance

Psychosocial Integrity

Physiological Integrity: Basic Care and Comfort, Pharmacological and Parenteral Therapies, Reduction of Risk Potential, and Physiological Adaptation

QUALITY AND SAFETY COMPETENCIES

Patient-Centered Care

Teamwork and Collaboration

Evidence-Based Practice

Quality Improvement

Safety

Informatics

Peer Review: _____   Faculty Review: _____

Grade Tracker

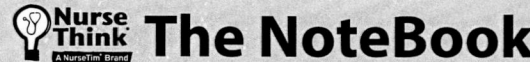
Related Concepts	**Related Exemplars/Diseases**

Reading/Resources - Clinical Judgment	**Class/Lab/Clinical – Clinical Judgment**

Priority Assessments or Cues	**Priority Labs & Diagnostics**	**Priority Nursing Interventions**
1	1	1
2	2	2
3	3	3

Priority Medications	**Priority Potential & Actual Complications**	**Priority Collaborative Goals**
1	1	1
2	2	2
3	3	3

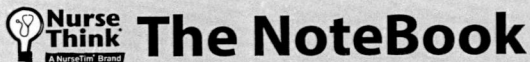
NurseThink® Quick

NEXT GEN LEARNING – NCLEX® TEST PLAN

Safe and Effective Care: Management of Care, Coordinated Care, Safety and Infection Control

Health Promotion and Maintenance

Psychosocial Integrity

Physiological Integrity: Basic Care and Comfort, Pharmacological and Parenteral Therapies, Reduction of Risk Potential, and Physiological Adaptation

QUALITY AND SAFETY COMPETENCIES

Patient-Centered Care

Teamwork and Collaboration

Evidence-Based Practice

Quality Improvement

Safety

Informatics

Peer Review: _____   Faculty Review: _____

Grade Tracker

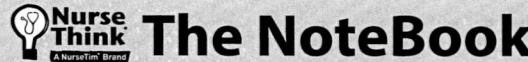
Related Concepts

Related Exemplars/Diseases

Reading/Resources - Clinical Judgment

Class/Lab/Clinical – Clinical Judgment

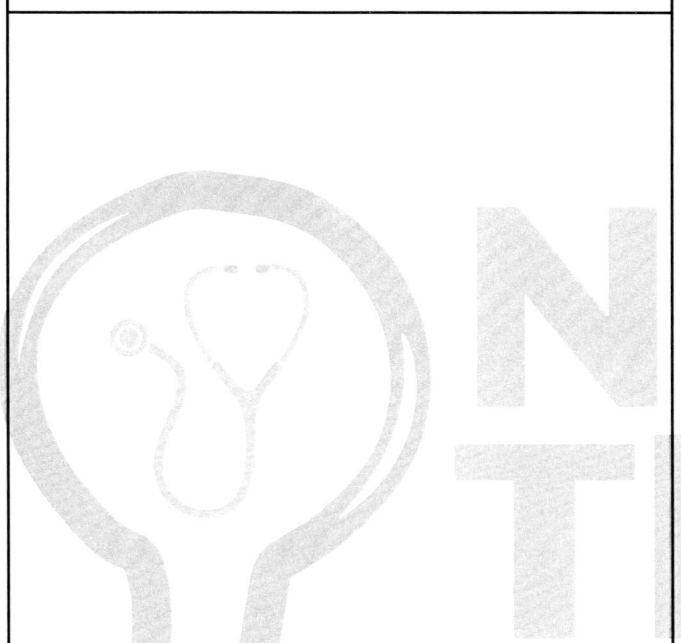

Priority Assessments or Cues

1

2

3

Priority Labs & Diagnostics

1

2

3

Priority Nursing Interventions

1

2

3

Priority Medications

1

2

3

Priority Potential & Actual Complications

1

2

3

Priority Collaborative Goals

1

2

3

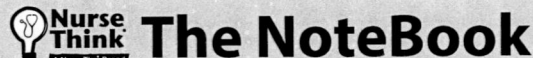

NurseThink® Quick

UTI- Causing Microorganisms

Keeps
Klebsiella
Enterococcus /Enterobacter
E-coli
Pseudomonas/Proteus mirabilis
Staphylococcus/Serratia

NEXT GEN LEARNING – NCLEX® TEST PLAN

Safe and Effective Care: Management of Care, Coordinated Care, Safety and Infection Control

Health Promotion and Maintenance

Psychosocial Integrity

Physiological Integrity: Basic Care and Comfort, Pharmacological and Parenteral Therapies, Reduction of Risk Potential, and Physiological Adaptation

QUALITY AND SAFETY COMPETENCIES

Patient-Centered Care

Teamwork and Collaboration

Evidence-Based Practice

Quality Improvement

Safety

Informatics

Peer Review: _____ Faculty Review: _____

Grade Tracker

Related Concepts	**Related Exemplars/Diseases**

Reading/Resources - Clinical Judgment	**Class/Lab/Clinical – Clinical Judgment**
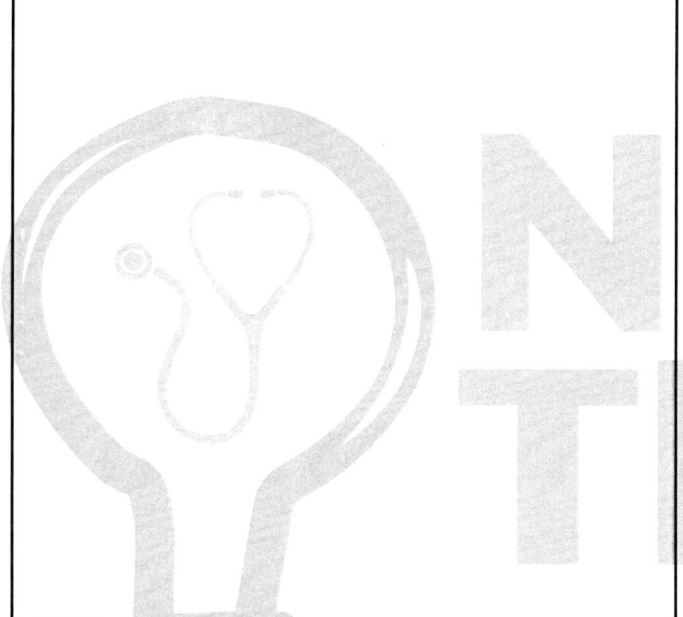	

Priority Assessments or Cues	**Priority Labs & Diagnostics**	**Priority Nursing Interventions**
1 2 3	1 2 3	1 2 3

Priority Medications	**Priority Potential & Actual Complications**	**Priority Collaborative Goals**
1 2 3	1 2 3	1 2 3

NurseThink® Quick

NEXT GEN LEARNING – NCLEX® TEST PLAN

Safe and Effective Care: Management of Care, Coordinated Care, Safety and Infection Control

Health Promotion and Maintenance

Psychosocial Integrity

Physiological Integrity: Basic Care and Comfort, Pharmacological and Parenteral Therapies, Reduction of Risk Potential, and Physiological Adaptation

QUALITY AND SAFETY COMPETENCIES

Patient-Centered Care

Teamwork and Collaboration

Evidence-Based Practice

Quality Improvement

Safety

Informatics

Peer Review: _____   Faculty Review: _____

Grade Tracker

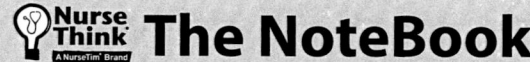

Related Concepts	**Related Exemplars/Diseases**

Reading/Resources - Clinical Judgment	**Class/Lab/Clinical – Clinical Judgment**

Priority Assessments or Cues	**Priority Labs & Diagnostics**	**Priority Nursing Interventions**
1	1	1
2	2	2
3	3	3

Priority Medications	**Priority Potential & Actual Complications**	**Priority Collaborative Goals**
1	1	1
2	2	2
3	3	3

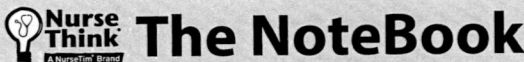
NurseThink® Quick

NEXT GEN LEARNING – NCLEX® TEST PLAN

Safe and Effective Care: Management of Care, Coordinated Care, Safety and Infection Control

Health Promotion and Maintenance

Psychosocial Integrity

Physiological Integrity: Basic Care and Comfort, Pharmacological and Parenteral Therapies, Reduction of Risk Potential, and Physiological Adaptation

QUALITY AND SAFETY COMPETENCIES

Patient-Centered Care

Teamwork and Collaboration

Evidence-Based Practice

Quality Improvement

Safety

Informatics

Peer Review: _____   Faculty Review: _____

Grade Tracker

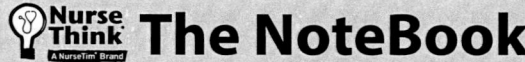
Related Concepts

Related Exemplars/Diseases

Reading/Resources - Clinical Judgment

Class/Lab/Clinical – Clinical Judgment

Priority Assessments or Cues

1

2

3

Priority Labs & Diagnostics

1

2

3

Priority Nursing Interventions

1

2

3

Priority Medications

1

2

3

Priority Potential & Actual Complications

1

2

3

Priority Collaborative Goals

1

2

3

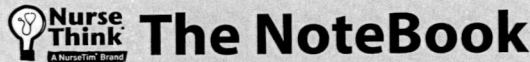
NurseThink® Quick

NEXT GEN LEARNING – NCLEX® TEST PLAN

Safe and Effective Care: Management of Care, Coordinated Care, Safety and Infection Control

Health Promotion and Maintenance

Psychosocial Integrity

Physiological Integrity: Basic Care and Comfort, Pharmacological and Parenteral Therapies, Reduction of Risk Potential, and Physiological Adaptation

QUALITY AND SAFETY COMPETENCIES

Patient-Centered Care

Teamwork and Collaboration

Evidence-Based Practice

Quality Improvement

Safety

Informatics

Peer Review: _____   Faculty Review: _____

Grade Tracker

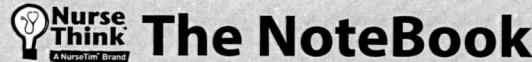
Related Concepts	Related Exemplars/Diseases

Reading/Resources - Clinical Judgment	Class/Lab/Clinical – Clinical Judgment

Priority Assessments or Cues	Priority Labs & Diagnostics	Priority Nursing Interventions
1	1	1
2	2	2
3	3	3

Priority Medications	Priority Potential & Actual Complications	Priority Collaborative Goals
1	1	1
2	2	2
3	3	3

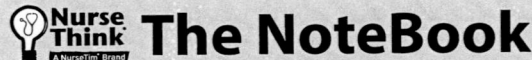

NurseThink® Quick

Pneumonia: Risk Factors
Inspiration
Immunosuppression
Neoplasia
Secretion retention
Pulmonary edema
Impaired alveolar macrophages
Respiratory infection, prior
Antibiotics & cytotoxics
Tracheal instrumentation
IV drug abuse
Other (general debility, immobility)
Neurologic impairment of cough reflex

NEXT GEN LEARNING – NCLEX® TEST PLAN

Safe and Effective Care: Management of Care, Coordinated Care, Safety and Infection Control

Health Promotion and Maintenance

Psychosocial Integrity

Physiological Integrity: Basic Care and Comfort, Pharmacological and Parenteral Therapies, Reduction of Risk Potential, and Physiological Adaptation

QUALITY AND SAFETY COMPETENCIES

Patient-Centered Care

Teamwork and Collaboration

Evidence-Based Practice

Quality Improvement

Safety

Informatics

Peer Review: _____   Faculty Review: _____

Grade Tracker

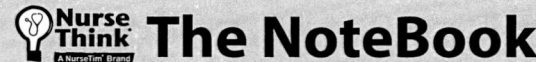
Related Concepts	Related Exemplars/Diseases

Reading/Resources - Clinical Judgment	Class/Lab/Clinical – Clinical Judgment

Priority Assessments or Cues

1

2

3

Priority Labs & Diagnostics

1

2

3

Priority Nursing Interventions

1

2

3

Priority Medications

1

2

3

Priority Potential & Actual Complications

1

2

3

Priority Collaborative Goals

1

2

3

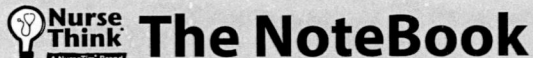
NurseThink® Quick

Anti-TB Drugs and Side Effects

Ripes
Rifampicin – red-orange urine
Isoniazid – peripheral neuritis
Pyrazinamide – increased uric acid
Ethambutol – eye problems
Streptomycin – ototoxic

NEXT GEN LEARNING – NCLEX® TEST PLAN

Safe and Effective Care: Management of Care, Coordinated Care, Safety and Infection Control

Health Promotion and Maintenance

Psychosocial Integrity

Physiological Integrity: Basic Care and Comfort, Pharmacological and Parenteral Therapies, Reduction of Risk Potential, and Physiological Adaptation

QUALITY AND SAFETY COMPETENCIES

Patient-Centered Care

Teamwork and Collaboration

Evidence-Based Practice

Quality Improvement

Safety

Informatics

Peer Review: _____   Faculty Review: _____

Grade Tracker

Related Concepts

Related Exemplars/Diseases

Reading/Resources - Clinical Judgment

Class/Lab/Clinical – Clinical Judgment

Priority Assessments or Cues
1
2
3

Priority Labs & Diagnostics
1
2
3

Priority Nursing Interventions
1
2
3

Priority Medications
1
2
3

Priority Potential & Actual Complications
1
2
3

Priority Collaborative Goals
1
2
3

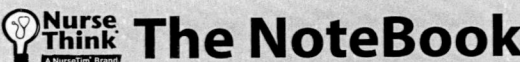
NurseThink® Quick

NEXT GEN LEARNING – NCLEX® TEST PLAN

Safe and Effective Care: Management of Care, Coordinated Care, Safety and Infection Control

Health Promotion and Maintenance

Psychosocial Integrity

Physiological Integrity: Basic Care and Comfort, Pharmacological and Parenteral Therapies, Reduction of Risk Potential, and Physiological Adaptation

QUALITY AND SAFETY COMPETENCIES

Patient-Centered Care

Teamwork and Collaboration

Evidence-Based Practice

Quality Improvement

Safety

Informatics

Peer Review: _____   Faculty Review: _____

Grade Tracker

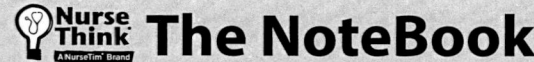

Related Concepts	Related Exemplars/Diseases

Reading/Resources - Clinical Judgment	Class/Lab/Clinical – Clinical Judgment

Priority Assessments or Cues	Priority Labs & Diagnostics	Priority Nursing Interventions
1	1	1
2	2	2
3	3	3

Priority Medications	Priority Potential & Actual Complications	Priority Collaborative Goals
1	1	1
2	2	2
3	3	3

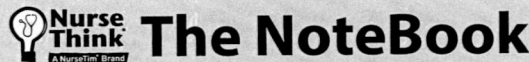
NurseThink® Quick

NEXT GEN LEARNING – NCLEX® TEST PLAN

Safe and Effective Care: Management of Care, Coordinated Care, Safety and Infection Control

Health Promotion and Maintenance

Psychosocial Integrity

Physiological Integrity: Basic Care and Comfort, Pharmacological and Parenteral Therapies, Reduction of Risk Potential, and Physiological Adaptation

QUALITY AND SAFETY COMPETENCIES

Patient-Centered Care

Teamwork and Collaboration

Evidence-Based Practice

Quality Improvement

Safety

Informatics

Peer Review: _____   Faculty Review: _____

Grade Tracker

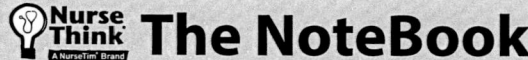

Related Concepts

Related Exemplars/Diseases

Reading/Resources - Clinical Judgment

Class/Lab/Clinical – Clinical Judgment

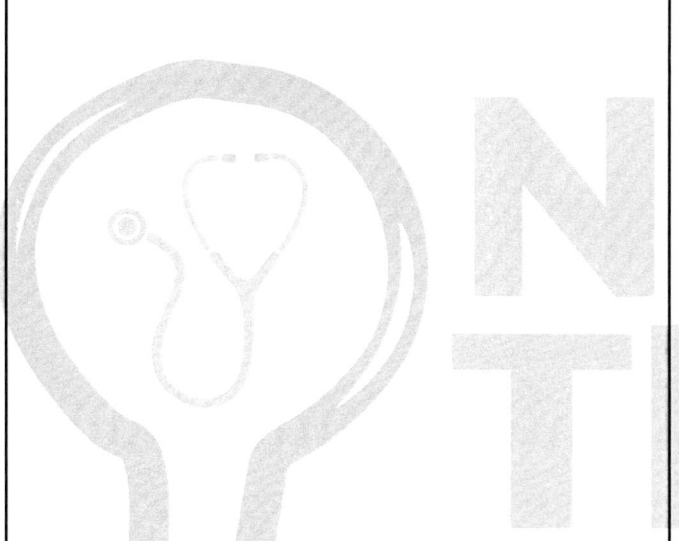

Priority Assessments or Cues

1

2

3

Priority Labs & Diagnostics

1

2

3

Priority Nursing Interventions

1

2

3

Priority Medications

1

2

3

Priority Potential & Actual Complications

1

2

3

Priority Collaborative Goals

1

2

3

NurseThink® Quick

Anti-Gout Medications	Gout: Precipitating Factors	Gout: Major Features
Cap Die	**Dark**	**Gout**
Colchicine - **D**eposition of uric acid	**D**iuretics	**G**reat toe
Allopurinol - **I**nhibits uric acid	**A**lcohol	**O**ne joint
Probenecid - **E**xcretion of uric acid	**R**enal disease	**U**ric acid increased
	Kicked (trauma)	**T**ophi

NEXT GEN LEARNING – NCLEX® TEST PLAN

Safe and Effective Care: Management of Care, Coordinated Care, Safety and Infection Control

Health Promotion and Maintenance

Psychosocial Integrity

Physiological Integrity: Basic Care and Comfort, Pharmacological and Parenteral Therapies, Reduction of Risk Potential, and Physiological Adaptation

QUALITY AND SAFETY COMPETENCIES

Patient-Centered Care

Teamwork and Collaboration

Evidence-Based Practice

Quality Improvement

Safety

Informatics

Peer Review: _____   Faculty Review: _____

Grade Tracker

Related Concepts

Related Exemplars/Diseases

Reading/Resources - Clinical Judgment

Class/Lab/Clinical – Clinical Judgment

Priority Assessments or Cues

1

2

3

Priority Labs & Diagnostics

1

2

3

Priority Nursing Interventions

1

2

3

Priority Medications

1

2

3

Priority Potential & Actual Complications

1

2

3

Priority Collaborative Goals

1

2

3

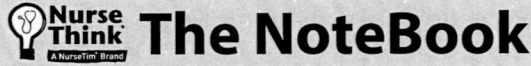
NurseThink® Quick

NEXT GEN LEARNING – NCLEX® TEST PLAN

Safe and Effective Care: Management of Care, Coordinated Care, Safety and Infection Control

Health Promotion and Maintenance

Psychosocial Integrity

Physiological Integrity: Basic Care and Comfort, Pharmacological and Parenteral Therapies, Reduction of Risk Potential, and Physiological Adaptation

QUALITY AND SAFETY COMPETENCIES

Patient-Centered Care

Teamwork and Collaboration

Evidence-Based Practice

Quality Improvement

Safety

Informatics

Peer Review: _____   Faculty Review: _____

Grade Tracker

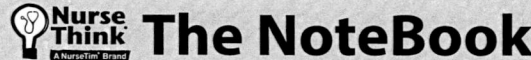
Related Concepts	Related Exemplars/Diseases

Reading/Resources - Clinical Judgment	Class/Lab/Clinical – Clinical Judgment

Priority Assessments or Cues	Priority Labs & Diagnostics	Priority Nursing Interventions
1	1	1
2	2	2
3	3	3

Priority Medications	Priority Potential & Actual Complications	Priority Collaborative Goals
1	1	1
2	2	2
3	3	3

NurseThink® Quick

NEXT GEN LEARNING – NCLEX® TEST PLAN

Safe and Effective Care: Management of Care, Coordinated Care, Safety and Infection Control

Health Promotion and Maintenance

Psychosocial Integrity

Physiological Integrity: Basic Care and Comfort, Pharmacological and Parenteral Therapies, Reduction of Risk Potential, and Physiological Adaptation

QUALITY AND SAFETY COMPETENCIES

Patient-Centered Care

Teamwork and Collaboration

Evidence-Based Practice

Quality Improvement

Safety

Informatics

Peer Review: _____   Faculty Review: _____

Grade Tracker

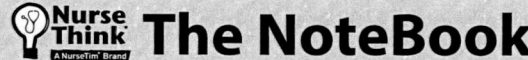
Related Concepts

Related Exemplars/Diseases

Reading/Resources - Clinical Judgment

Class/Lab/Clinical – Clinical Judgment

Priority Assessments or Cues

1

2

3

Priority Labs & Diagnostics

1

2

3

Priority Nursing Interventions

1

2

3

Priority Medications

1

2

3

Priority Potential & Actual Complications

1

2

3

Priority Collaborative Goals

1

2

3

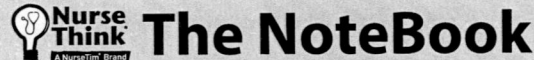

NurseThink® Quick

Polycythemia Rubra Vera: Symptoms

PRV
Plethora/Pruritus
Ringing in ears
Visual blurriness

NEXT GEN LEARNING – NCLEX® TEST PLAN

Safe and Effective Care: Management of Care, Coordinated Care, Safety and Infection Control

Health Promotion and Maintenance

Psychosocial Integrity

Physiological Integrity: Basic Care and Comfort, Pharmacological and Parenteral Therapies, Reduction of Risk Potential, and Physiological Adaptation

QUALITY AND SAFETY COMPETENCIES

Patient-Centered Care

Teamwork and Collaboration

Evidence-Based Practice

Quality Improvement

Safety

Informatics

Peer Review: _____   Faculty Review: _____

Grade Tracker

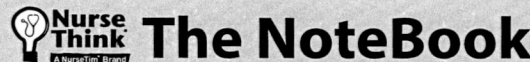
Related Concepts

Related Exemplars/Diseases

Reading/Resources - Clinical Judgment

Class/Lab/Clinical – Clinical Judgment

Priority Assessments or Cues

1

2

3

Priority Labs & Diagnostics

1

2

3

Priority Nursing Interventions

1

2

3

Priority Medications

1

2

3

Priority Potential & Actual Complications

1

2

3

Priority Collaborative Goals

1

2

3

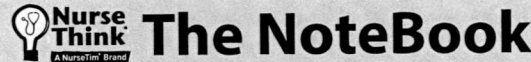
NurseThink® Quick

<table>
<tr><td></td><td></td><td></td></tr>
</table>

NEXT GEN LEARNING – NCLEX® TEST PLAN

Safe and Effective Care: Management of Care, Coordinated Care, Safety and Infection Control

Health Promotion and Maintenance

Psychosocial Integrity

Physiological Integrity: Basic Care and Comfort, Pharmacological and Parenteral Therapies, Reduction of Risk Potential, and Physiological Adaptation

QUALITY AND SAFETY COMPETENCIES

Patient-Centered Care

Teamwork and Collaboration

Evidence-Based Practice

Quality Improvement

Safety

Informatics

Peer Review: _____   Faculty Review: _____

Grade Tracker

<table>
<tr><td></td><td></td><td></td><td></td><td></td><td></td><td></td><td></td><td></td><td></td><td></td><td></td><td></td><td></td><td></td><td></td></tr>
</table>

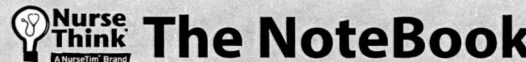

Related Concepts

Related Exemplars/Diseases

Reading/Resources - Clinical Judgment

Class/Lab/Clinical – Clinical Judgment

Priority Assessments or Cues

1

2

3

Priority Labs & Diagnostics

1

2

3

Priority Nursing Interventions

1

2

3

Priority Medications

1

2

3

Priority Potential & Actual Complications

1

2

3

Priority Collaborative Goals

1

2

3

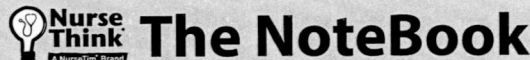

NurseThink® Quick

Bleeding Disorders: Signs and Symptoms

Beep
Bleeding gums
Ecchymosis (bruises)
Epistaxis (nosebleed)
Petechiae (tiny purplish spots)

Thrombotic Thrombocytopenic Purpura: Signs

Fat RN
Fever
Anemia
Thrombocytopenia
Renal problems
Neurologic dysfunction

TTP: Clinical Features

Partner
Platelet count low
Anemia
Renal failure
Temperature rise
Neurological deficits
ER admission

NEXT GEN LEARNING – NCLEX® TEST PLAN

Safe and Effective Care: Management of Care, Coordinated Care, Safety and Infection Control

Health Promotion and Maintenance

Psychosocial Integrity

Physiological Integrity: Basic Care and Comfort, Pharmacological and Parenteral Therapies, Reduction of Risk Potential, and Physiological Adaptation

QUALITY AND SAFETY COMPETENCIES

Patient-Centered Care

Teamwork and Collaboration

Evidence-Based Practice

Quality Improvement

Safety

Informatics

Peer Review: _____   Faculty Review: _____

Grade Tracker

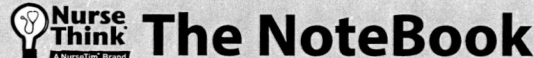
Related Concepts	**Related Exemplars/Diseases**

Reading/Resources - Clinical Judgment	**Class/Lab/Clinical – Clinical Judgment**

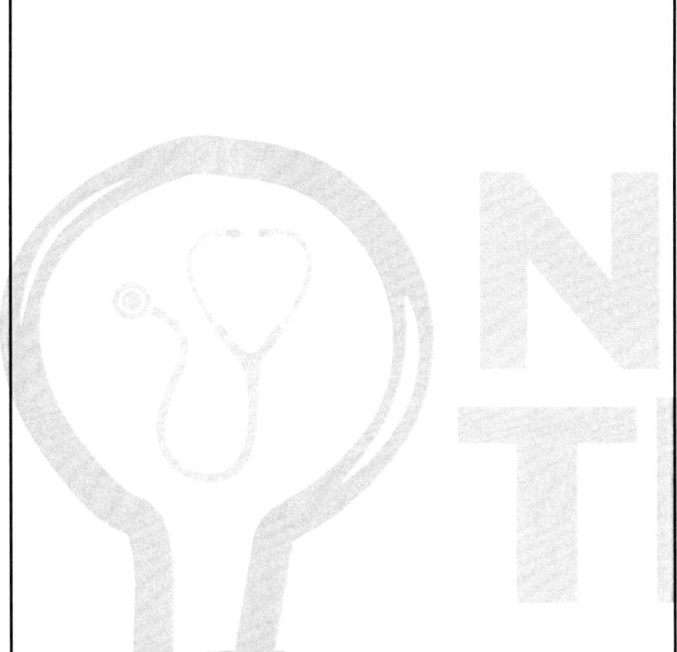

Priority Assessments or Cues	**Priority Labs & Diagnostics**	**Priority Nursing Interventions**
1	1	1
2	2	2
3	3	3

Priority Medications	**Priority Potential & Actual Complications**	**Priority Collaborative Goals**
1	1	1
2	2	2
3	3	3

NurseThink® Quick

NEXT GEN LEARNING – NCLEX® TEST PLAN

Safe and Effective Care: Management of Care, Coordinated Care, Safety and Infection Control

Health Promotion and Maintenance

Psychosocial Integrity

Physiological Integrity: Basic Care and Comfort, Pharmacological and Parenteral Therapies, Reduction of Risk Potential, and Physiological Adaptation

QUALITY AND SAFETY COMPETENCIES

Patient-Centered Care

Teamwork and Collaboration

Evidence-Based Practice

Quality Improvement

Safety

Informatics

Peer Review: _____ Faculty Review: _____

Grade Tracker

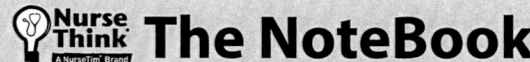
Related Concepts

Related Exemplars/Diseases

Reading/Resources - Clinical Judgment

Class/Lab/Clinical – Clinical Judgment

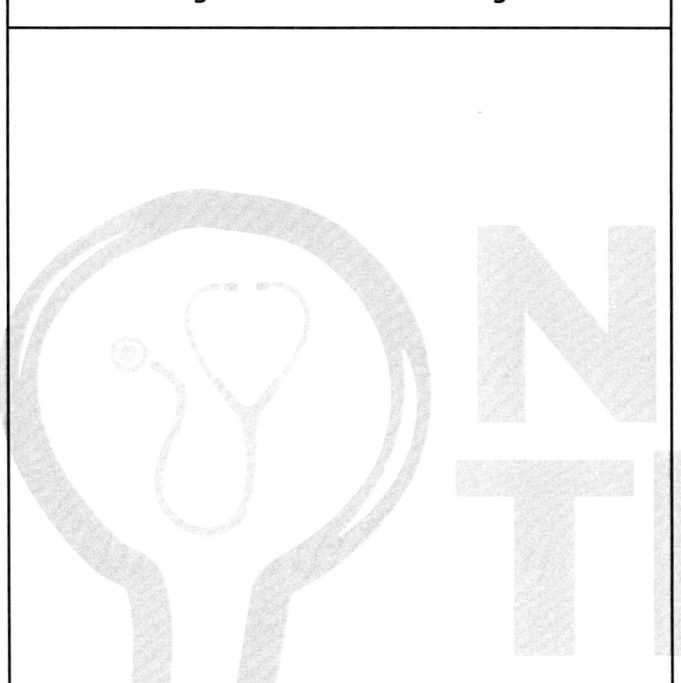

Priority Assessments or Cues

1

2

3

Priority Labs & Diagnostics

1

2

3

Priority Nursing Interventions

1

2

3

Priority Medications

1

2

3

Priority Potential & Actual Complications

1

2

3

Priority Collaborative Goals

1

2

3

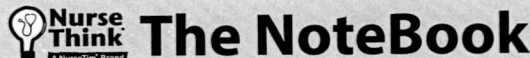

NurseThink® Quick

Carcinomas that Metastasize to Bone		
Carcinomas that Metastasize to Bone		
Particular Tumors Love Killing Bone		
Prostate		
Thyroid		
Lung		
Kidney		
Breast		

NEXT GEN LEARNING – NCLEX® TEST PLAN

Safe and Effective Care: Management of Care, Coordinated Care, Safety and Infection Control

Health Promotion and Maintenance

Psychosocial Integrity

Physiological Integrity: Basic Care and Comfort, Pharmacological and Parenteral Therapies, Reduction of Risk Potential, and Physiological Adaptation

QUALITY AND SAFETY COMPETENCIES

Patient-Centered Care

Teamwork and Collaboration

Evidence-Based Practice

Quality Improvement

Safety

Informatics

Peer Review: _____   Faculty Review: _____

Grade Tracker

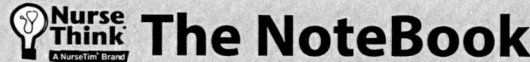

Related Concepts	Related Exemplars/Diseases

Reading/Resources - Clinical Judgment	Class/Lab/Clinical – Clinical Judgment

Priority Assessments or Cues	Priority Labs & Diagnostics	Priority Nursing Interventions
1	1	1
2	2	2
3	3	3

Priority Medications	Priority Potential & Actual Complications	Priority Collaborative Goals
1	1	1
2	2	2
3	3	3

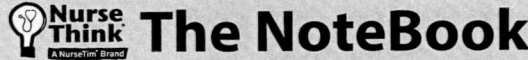
NurseThink® Quick

NEXT GEN LEARNING – NCLEX® TEST PLAN

Safe and Effective Care: Management of Care, Coordinated Care, Safety and Infection Control

Health Promotion and Maintenance

Psychosocial Integrity

Physiological Integrity: Basic Care and Comfort, Pharmacological and Parenteral Therapies, Reduction of Risk Potential, and Physiological Adaptation

QUALITY AND SAFETY COMPETENCIES

Patient-Centered Care

Teamwork and Collaboration

Evidence-Based Practice

Quality Improvement

Safety

Informatics

Peer Review: _____   Faculty Review: _____

Grade Tracker

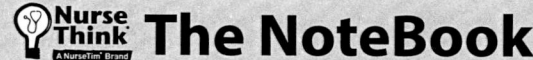
Related Concepts	**Related Exemplars/Diseases**

Reading/Resources - Clinical Judgment	**Class/Lab/Clinical – Clinical Judgment**

Priority Assessments or Cues	**Priority Labs & Diagnostics**	**Priority Nursing Interventions**
1	1	1
2	2	2
3	3	3

Priority Medications	**Priority Potential & Actual Complications**	**Priority Collaborative Goals**
1	1	1
2	2	2
3	3	3

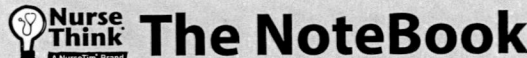
NurseThink® Quick

Breast Self-Examination Song
Tune of 3 little Indians

♫ ♪ ♪ ♫ 1 little 2, little 3 little fingers Do BSE 7 days after menses
Press nipple once for discharge, call your doctor
I'm sure you will do it more...♫ ♪ ♪

NEXT GEN LEARNING – NCLEX® TEST PLAN

Safe and Effective Care: Management of Care, Coordinated Care, Safety and Infection Control

Health Promotion and Maintenance

Psychosocial Integrity

Physiological Integrity: Basic Care and Comfort, Pharmacological and Parenteral Therapies, Reduction of Risk Potential, and Physiological Adaptation

QUALITY AND SAFETY COMPETENCIES

Patient-Centered Care

Teamwork and Collaboration

Evidence-Based Practice

Quality Improvement

Safety

Informatics

Peer Review: _____   Faculty Review: _____

Grade Tracker

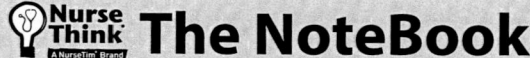
Related Concepts	Related Exemplars/Diseases

Reading/Resources - Clinical Judgment	Class/Lab/Clinical – Clinical Judgment

Priority Assessments or Cues
1
2
3

Priority Labs & Diagnostics
1
2
3

Priority Nursing Interventions
1
2
3

Priority Medications
1

2

3

Priority Potential & Actual Complications
1

2

3

Priority Collaborative Goals
1

2

3

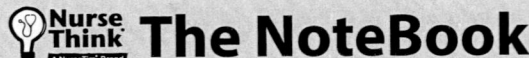
NurseThink® Quick

Colon Carcinoma: Causes	Colon Cancer: Risk Factors	
Craps	**Hula**	
Chronic ulcerative colitis	**H**eredity/Hereditary diseases	
Ratio of animal fat to fiber diet A – Adenomatous polyps	**U**lcerative colitis	
Polyposis (Familial)	**L**ow-fiber, high-fat diet	
Strong family history of colon cancer	**A**denomatous polyps	

NEXT GEN LEARNING – NCLEX® TEST PLAN

Safe and Effective Care: Management of Care, Coordinated Care, Safety and Infection Control

Health Promotion and Maintenance

Psychosocial Integrity

Physiological Integrity: Basic Care and Comfort, Pharmacological and Parenteral Therapies, Reduction of Risk Potential, and Physiological Adaptation

QUALITY AND SAFETY COMPETENCIES

Patient-Centered Care

Teamwork and Collaboration

Evidence-Based Practice

Quality Improvement

Safety

Informatics

Peer Review: _____   Faculty Review: _____

Grade Tracker

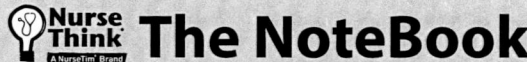

Related Concepts	Related Exemplars/Diseases

Reading/Resources - Clinical Judgment	Class/Lab/Clinical – Clinical Judgment
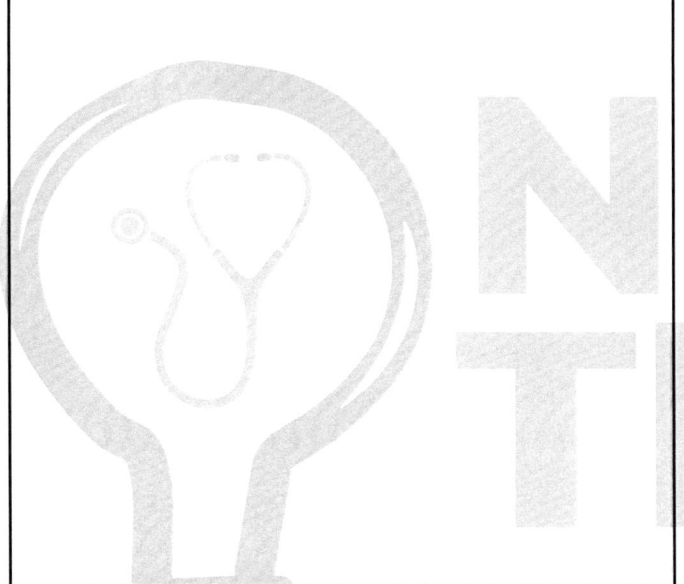	

Priority Assessments or Cues	Priority Labs & Diagnostics	Priority Nursing Interventions
1	1	1
2	2	2
3	3	3

Priority Medications	Priority Potential & Actual Complications	Priority Collaborative Goals
1	1	1
2	2	2
3	3	3

NurseThink® Quick

Safe and Effective Care: Management of Care, Coordinated Care, Safety and Infection Control

Health Promotion and Maintenance

Psychosocial Integrity

Physiological Integrity: Basic Care and Comfort, Pharmacological and Parenteral Therapies, Reduction of Risk Potential, and Physiological Adaptation

QUALITY AND SAFETY COMPETENCIES

Patient-Centered Care

Teamwork and Collaboration

Evidence-Based Practice

Quality Improvement

Safety

Informatics

Peer Review: _____   Faculty Review: _____

Grade Tracker

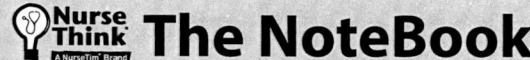
Related Concepts

Related Exemplars/Diseases

Reading/Resources - Clinical Judgment

Class/Lab/Clinical – Clinical Judgment

Priority Assessments or Cues
1
2
3

Priority Labs & Diagnostics
1
2
3

Priority Nursing Interventions
1
2
3

Priority Medications
1
2
3

Priority Potential & Actual Complications
1
2
3

Priority Collaborative Goals
1
2
3

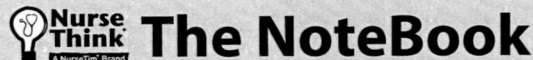
NurseThink® Quick

NEXT GEN LEARNING – NCLEX® TEST PLAN

Safe and Effective Care: Management of Care, Coordinated Care, Safety and Infection Control

Health Promotion and Maintenance

Psychosocial Integrity

Physiological Integrity: Basic Care and Comfort, Pharmacological and Parenteral Therapies, Reduction of Risk Potential, and Physiological Adaptation

QUALITY AND SAFETY COMPETENCIES

Patient-Centered Care

Teamwork and Collaboration

Evidence-Based Practice

Quality Improvement

Safety

Informatics

Peer Review: _____   Faculty Review: _____

Grade Tracker

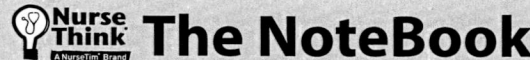
Related Concepts	Related Exemplars/Diseases

Reading/Resources - Clinical Judgment	Class/Lab/Clinical – Clinical Judgment
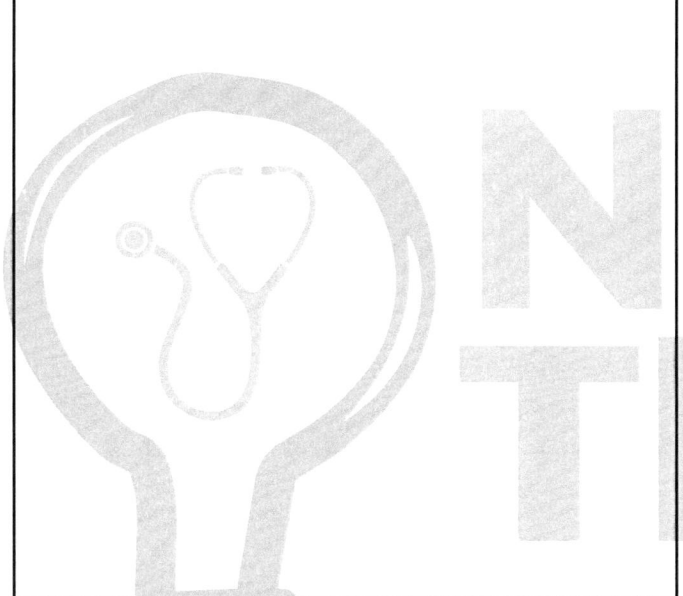	

Priority Assessments or Cues
1
2
3

Priority Labs & Diagnostics
1
2
3

Priority Nursing Interventions
1
2
3

Priority Medications
1
2
3

Priority Potential & Actual Complications
1
2
3

Priority Collaborative Goals
1
2
3

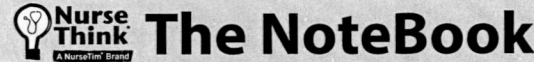
NurseThink® Quick

NEXT GEN LEARNING – NCLEX® TEST PLAN

Safe and Effective Care: Management of Care, Coordinated Care, Safety and Infection Control

Health Promotion and Maintenance

Psychosocial Integrity

Physiological Integrity: Basic Care and Comfort, Pharmacological and Parenteral Therapies, Reduction of Risk Potential, and Physiological Adaptation

QUALITY AND SAFETY COMPETENCIES

Patient-Centered Care

Teamwork and Collaboration

Evidence-Based Practice

Quality Improvement

Safety

Informatics

Peer Review: _____   Faculty Review: _____

Grade Tracker

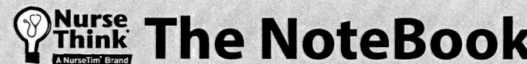

Related Concepts	**Related Exemplars/Diseases**

Reading/Resources - Clinical Judgment	**Class/Lab/Clinical – Clinical Judgment**

Priority Assessments or Cues	**Priority Labs & Diagnostics**	**Priority Nursing Interventions**
1	1	1
2	2	2
3	3	3

Priority Medications	**Priority Potential & Actual Complications**	**Priority Collaborative Goals**
1	1	1
2	2	2
3	3	3

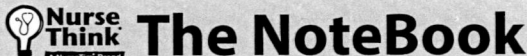
NurseThink® Quick

Lymphoma: Staging of B-Cell CLL (RAI) ***LOATh*** I: **L**ymphadenopathy II: **O**rganomegaly (splenomegaly) III: **A**nemia IV: **Th**rombocytopenia		

NEXT GEN LEARNING – NCLEX® TEST PLAN

Safe and Effective Care: Management of Care, Coordinated Care, Safety and Infection Control

Health Promotion and Maintenance

Psychosocial Integrity

Physiological Integrity: Basic Care and Comfort, Pharmacological and Parenteral Therapies, Reduction of Risk Potential, and Physiological Adaptation

QUALITY AND SAFETY COMPETENCIES

Patient-Centered Care

Teamwork and Collaboration

Evidence-Based Practice

Quality Improvement

Safety

Informatics

Peer Review: _____   Faculty Review: _____

Grade Tracker

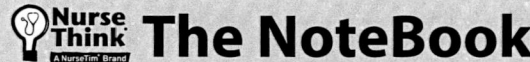
Related Concepts	Related Exemplars/Diseases

Reading/Resources - Clinical Judgment	Class/Lab/Clinical – Clinical Judgment

Priority Assessments or Cues

1

2

3

Priority Labs & Diagnostics

1

2

3

Priority Nursing Interventions

1

2

3

Priority Medications

1

2

3

Priority Potential & Actual Complications

1

2

3

Priority Collaborative Goals

1

2

3

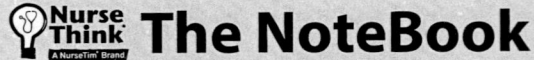
NurseThink® Quick

Multiple Myeloma: Symptoms *BAHRAIN UV* **B**one Pain **A**nemia **H**ypercalcemia **R**enal failure **A**myloidosis **I**nfection **N**europathy **U**ricaemia **V**iscosity		

NEXT GEN LEARNING – NCLEX® TEST PLAN

Safe and Effective Care: Management of Care, Coordinated Care, Safety and Infection Control

Health Promotion and Maintenance

Psychosocial Integrity

Physiological Integrity: Basic Care and Comfort, Pharmacological and Parenteral Therapies, Reduction of Risk Potential, and Physiological Adaptation

QUALITY AND SAFETY COMPETENCIES

Patient-Centered Care

Teamwork and Collaboration

Evidence-Based Practice

Quality Improvement

Safety

Informatics

Peer Review: _____   Faculty Review: _____

Grade Tracker

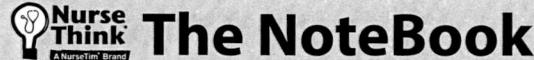
Related Concepts

Related Exemplars/Diseases

Reading/Resources - Clinical Judgment

Class/Lab/Clinical – Clinical Judgment

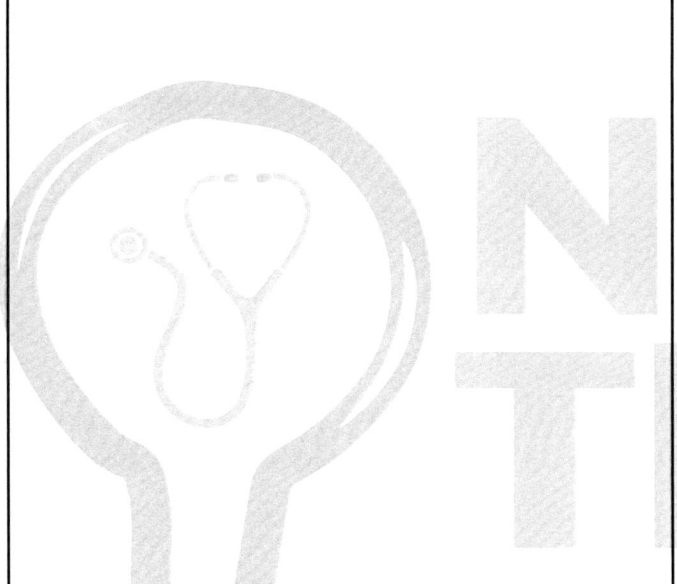

Priority Assessments or Cues

1

2

3

Priority Labs & Diagnostics

1

2

3

Priority Nursing Interventions

1

2

3

Priority Medications

1

2

3

Priority Potential & Actual Complications

1

2

3

Priority Collaborative Goals

1

2

3

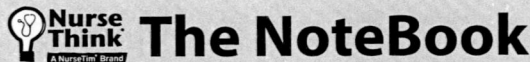
NurseThink® Quick

NEXT GEN LEARNING – NCLEX® TEST PLAN

Safe and Effective Care: Management of Care, Coordinated Care, Safety and Infection Control

Health Promotion and Maintenance

Psychosocial Integrity

Physiological Integrity: Basic Care and Comfort, Pharmacological and Parenteral Therapies, Reduction of Risk Potential, and Physiological Adaptation

QUALITY AND SAFETY COMPETENCIES

Patient-Centered Care

Teamwork and Collaboration

Evidence-Based Practice

Quality Improvement

Safety

Informatics

Peer Review: _____   Faculty Review: _____

Grade Tracker

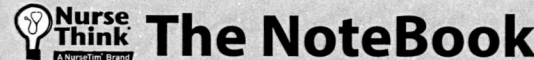
Related Concepts	Related Exemplars/Diseases

Reading/Resources - Clinical Judgment	Class/Lab/Clinical – Clinical Judgment
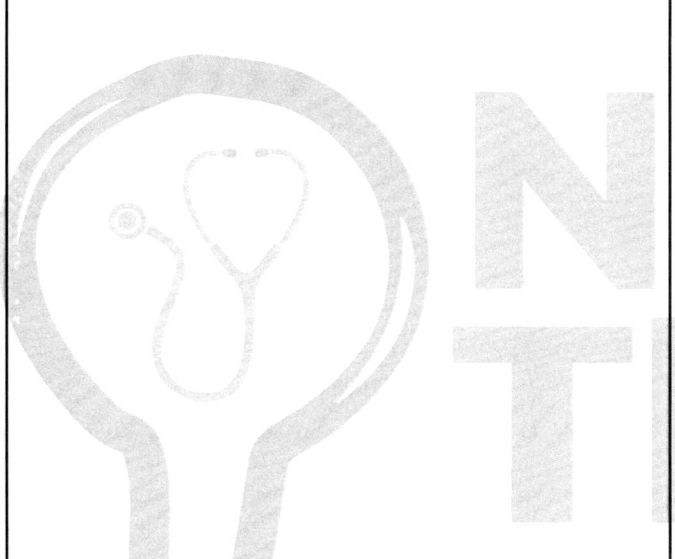	

Priority Assessments or Cues
1
2
3

Priority Labs & Diagnostics
1
2
3

Priority Nursing Interventions
1
2
3

Priority Medications
1
2
3

Priority Potential & Actual Complications
1
2
3

Priority Collaborative Goals
1
2
3

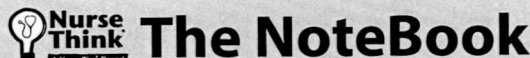
NurseThink® Quick

Malignant Mole: Signs and Symptoms ***ABCD*** **A**symmetry: is the mole irregular in shape? **B**order: is the border irregular, notched, or poorly defined? **C**olor: does the color vary **D**iameter: is the diameter more than 6 mm?	**Malignant Melanoma: 3 sites with poor prognosis** ***Bans*** **B**ack of arm **N**eck **S**calp	

NEXT GEN LEARNING – NCLEX® TEST PLAN

Safe and Effective Care: Management of Care, Coordinated Care, Safety and Infection Control

Health Promotion and Maintenance

Psychosocial Integrity

Physiological Integrity: Basic Care and Comfort, Pharmacological and Parenteral Therapies, Reduction of Risk Potential, and Physiological Adaptation

QUALITY AND SAFETY COMPETENCIES

Patient-Centered Care

Teamwork and Collaboration

Evidence-Based Practice

Quality Improvement

Safety

Informatics

Peer Review: _____   Faculty Review: _____

Grade Tracker

Related Concepts

Related Exemplars/Diseases

Reading/Resources - Clinical Judgment

Class/Lab/Clinical – Clinical Judgment

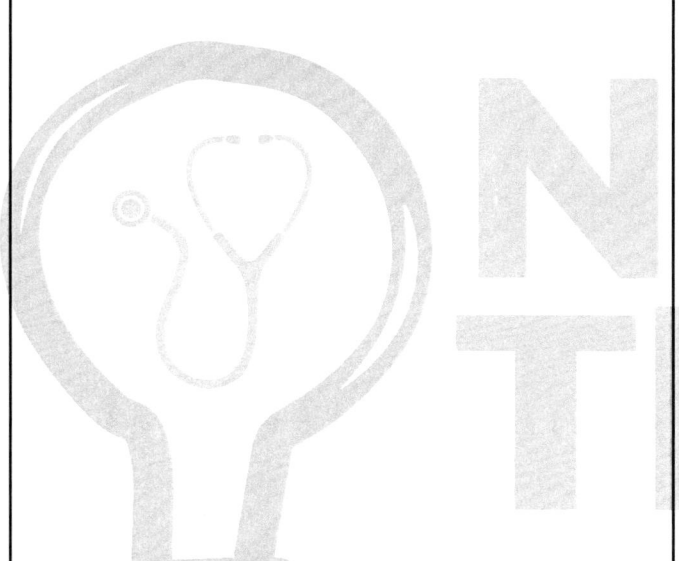

Priority Assessments or Cues

1
2
3

Priority Labs & Diagnostics

1
2
3

Priority Nursing Interventions

1
2
3

Priority Medications

1

2

3

Priority Potential & Actual Complications

1

2

3

Priority Collaborative Goals

1

2

3

NurseThink® Quick

ICP waveforms	Increased ICP: Cushing's Triad	
ABC's	**Hyper-Brady-Brady**	
A is Awful	**Hypertension** (wise pulse pressure)	
B is Bad	**Bradycardia**	
C is Common	**Bradypnea**	

NEXT GEN LEARNING – NCLEX® TEST PLAN

Safe and Effective Care: Management of Care, Coordinated Care, Safety and Infection Control

Health Promotion and Maintenance

Psychosocial Integrity

Physiological Integrity: Basic Care and Comfort, Pharmacological and Parenteral Therapies, Reduction of Risk Potential, and Physiological Adaptation

QUALITY AND SAFETY COMPETENCIES

Patient-Centered Care

Teamwork and Collaboration

Evidence-Based Practice

Quality Improvement

Safety

Informatics

Peer Review: _____   Faculty Review: _____

Grade Tracker

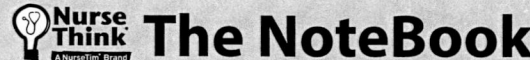

Related Concepts	Related Exemplars/Diseases

Reading/Resources - Clinical Judgment	Class/Lab/Clinical – Clinical Judgment

Priority Assessments or Cues	Priority Labs & Diagnostics	Priority Nursing Interventions
1	1	1
2	2	2
3	3	3

Priority Medications	Priority Potential & Actual Complications	Priority Collaborative Goals
1	1	1
2	2	2
3	3	3

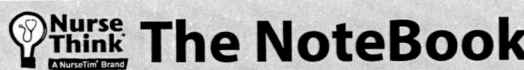
NurseThink® Quick

NEXT GEN LEARNING – NCLEX® TEST PLAN

Safe and Effective Care: Management of Care, Coordinated Care, Safety and Infection Control

Health Promotion and Maintenance

Psychosocial Integrity

Physiological Integrity: Basic Care and Comfort, Pharmacological and Parenteral Therapies, Reduction of Risk Potential, and Physiological Adaptation

QUALITY AND SAFETY COMPETENCIES

Patient-Centered Care

Teamwork and Collaboration

Evidence-Based Practice

Quality Improvement

Safety

Informatics

Peer Review: _____   Faculty Review: _____

Grade Tracker

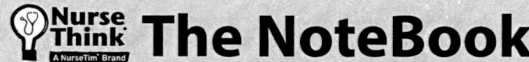
Related Concepts

Related Exemplars/Diseases

Reading/Resources - Clinical Judgment

Class/Lab/Clinical – Clinical Judgment

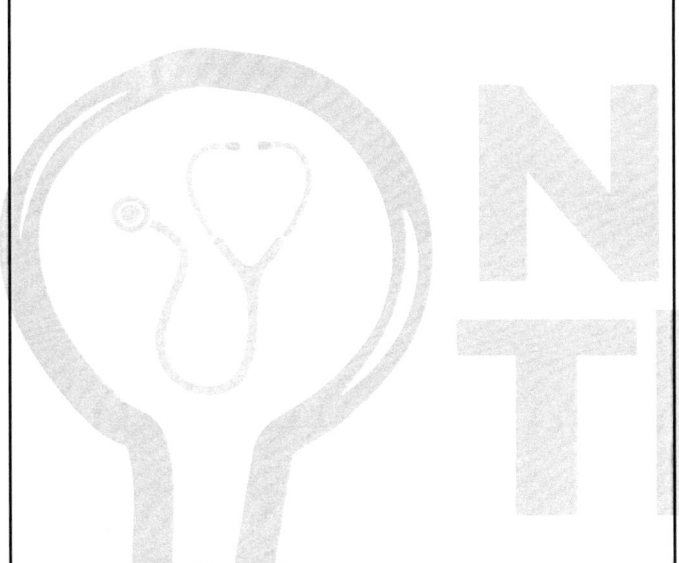

Priority Assessments or Cues

1

2

3

Priority Labs & Diagnostics

1

2

3

Priority Nursing Interventions

1

2

3

Priority Medications

1

2

3

Priority Potential & Actual Complications

1

2

3

Priority Collaborative Goals

1

2

3

NurseThink® Quick

NurseThink.com

NEXT GEN LEARNING – NCLEX® TEST PLAN

Safe and Effective Care: Management of Care, Coordinated Care, Safety and Infection Control

Health Promotion and Maintenance

Psychosocial Integrity

Physiological Integrity: Basic Care and Comfort, Pharmacological and Parenteral Therapies, Reduction of Risk Potential, and Physiological Adaptation

QUALITY AND SAFETY COMPETENCIES

Patient-Centered Care

Teamwork and Collaboration

Evidence-Based Practice

Quality Improvement

Safety

Informatics

Peer Review: _____   Faculty Review: _____

Grade Tracker

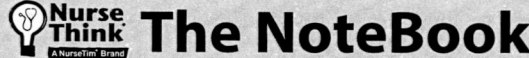
Related Concepts	Related Exemplars/Diseases

Reading/Resources - Clinical Judgment	Class/Lab/Clinical – Clinical Judgment

Priority Assessments or Cues

1
2
3

Priority Labs & Diagnostics

1
2
3

Priority Nursing Interventions

1
2
3

Priority Medications

1

2

3

Priority Potential & Actual Complications

1

2

3

Priority Collaborative Goals

1

2

3

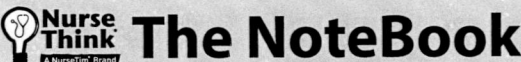

NurseThink® Quick

NEXT GEN LEARNING – NCLEX® TEST PLAN

Safe and Effective Care: Management of Care, Coordinated Care, Safety and Infection Control

Health Promotion and Maintenance

Psychosocial Integrity

Physiological Integrity: Basic Care and Comfort, Pharmacological and Parenteral Therapies, Reduction of Risk Potential, and Physiological Adaptation

QUALITY AND SAFETY COMPETENCIES

Patient-Centered Care

Teamwork and Collaboration

Evidence-Based Practice

Quality Improvement

Safety

Informatics

Peer Review: _____   Faculty Review: _____

Grade Tracker

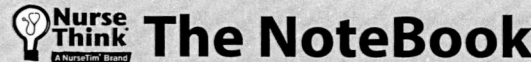
Related Concepts

Related Exemplars/Diseases

Reading/Resources - Clinical Judgment

Class/Lab/Clinical – Clinical Judgment

Priority Assessments or Cues

1

2

3

Priority Labs & Diagnostics

1

2

3

Priority Nursing Interventions

1

2

3

Priority Medications

1

2

3

Priority Potential & Actual Complications

1

2

3

Priority Collaborative Goals

1

2

3

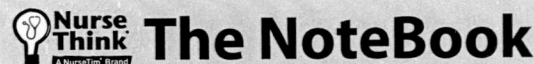
NurseThink® Quick

NEXT GEN LEARNING – NCLEX® TEST PLAN

Safe and Effective Care: Management of Care, Coordinated Care, Safety and Infection Control

Health Promotion and Maintenance

Psychosocial Integrity

Physiological Integrity: Basic Care and Comfort, Pharmacological and Parenteral Therapies, Reduction of Risk Potential, and Physiological Adaptation

QUALITY AND SAFETY COMPETENCIES

Patient-Centered Care

Teamwork and Collaboration

Evidence-Based Practice

Quality Improvement

Safety

Informatics

Peer Review: _____   Faculty Review: _____

Grade Tracker

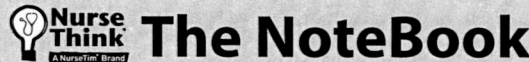

Related Concepts

Related Exemplars/Diseases

Reading/Resources - Clinical Judgment

Class/Lab/Clinical – Clinical Judgment

Priority Assessments or Cues

1

2

3

Priority Labs & Diagnostics

1

2

3

Priority Nursing Interventions

1

2

3

Priority Medications

1

2

3

Priority Potential & Actual Complications

1

2

3

Priority Collaborative Goals

1

2

3

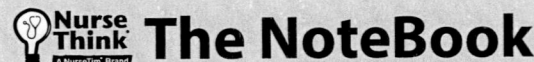
NurseThink® Quick

Hepatitis: Transmission Routes
Vowels are Bowels
   Hepatitis A and E transmitted by
   fecal- oral route

NEXT GEN LEARNING – NCLEX® TEST PLAN

Safe and Effective Care: Management of Care, Coordinated Care, Safety and Infection Control

Health Promotion and Maintenance

Psychosocial Integrity

Physiological Integrity: Basic Care and Comfort, Pharmacological and Parenteral Therapies, Reduction of Risk Potential, and Physiological Adaptation

QUALITY AND SAFETY COMPETENCIES

Patient-Centered Care

Teamwork and Collaboration

Evidence-Based Practice

Quality Improvement

Safety

Informatics

Peer Review: _____   Faculty Review: _____

Grade Tracker

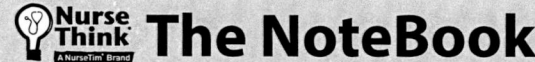

Related Concepts

Related Exemplars/Diseases

Reading/Resources - Clinical Judgment

Class/Lab/Clinical – Clinical Judgment

Priority Assessments or Cues
1
2
3

Priority Labs & Diagnostics
1
2
3

Priority Nursing Interventions
1
2
3

Priority Medications
1

2

3

Priority Potential & Actual Complications
1

2

3

Priority Collaborative Goals
1

2

3

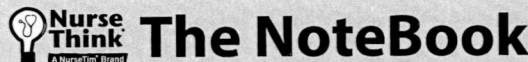
NurseThink® Quick

Hepatotoxic Drugs	Elevated ALT or AST Values	Liver Failure
8 A's and SGPT/SGOT	**ABCDEFGHIM**	**Claps**
Antituberculosis	**A**utoimmune hepatitis	**C**lubbing
Anticonvulsant	Hepatitis **B**	**L**eukonychia
Sodium luminal	Hepatitis **C**	**A**sterixis
Gabapentin	**D**rugs or toxins	**P**almar Erythema
Phenytoin	**E**thanol	**S**cratch marks
Tegretol	**F**atty liver	
Anticancer	**G**rowths of tumors	
Aspirin	**H**emodynamic disorder	
Alcohol	**I**ron or copper deficiency	
Antifamily (contraceptive pills)	**M**uscle Injury	
Acetaminophen		
Aflatoxins		

NEXT GEN LEARNING – NCLEX® TEST PLAN

Safe and Effective Care: Management of Care, Coordinated Care, Safety and Infection Control

Health Promotion and Maintenance

Psychosocial Integrity

Physiological Integrity: Basic Care and Comfort, Pharmacological and Parenteral Therapies, Reduction of Risk Potential, and Physiological Adaptation

QUALITY AND SAFETY COMPETENCIES

Patient-Centered Care

Teamwork and Collaboration

Evidence-Based Practice

Quality Improvement

Safety

Informatics

Peer Review: _____ Faculty Review: _____

Grade Tracker

Related Concepts

Related Exemplars/Diseases

Reading/Resources - Clinical Judgment

Class/Lab/Clinical – Clinical Judgment

Priority Assessments or Cues

1
2
3

Priority Labs & Diagnostics

1
2
3

Priority Nursing Interventions

1
2
3

Priority Medications

1
2
3

Priority Potential & Actual Complications

1
2
3

Priority Collaborative Goals

1
2
3

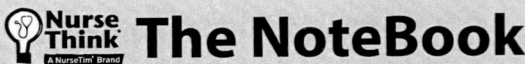
NurseThink® Quick

Addison's Causes *Antam* **A**utoimmune **N**eoplastic **T**B **A**myloid **M**eningococcal	President Kennedy had Addison's Disease: He always had a great tan. A President would need cortisol to respond to stress and hypoglycemia.	

NEXT GEN LEARNING – NCLEX® TEST PLAN

Safe and Effective Care: Management of Care, Coordinated Care, Safety and Infection Control

Health Promotion and Maintenance

Psychosocial Integrity

Physiological Integrity: Basic Care and Comfort, Pharmacological and Parenteral Therapies, Reduction of Risk Potential, and Physiological Adaptation

QUALITY AND SAFETY COMPETENCIES

Patient-Centered Care

Teamwork and Collaboration

Evidence-Based Practice

Quality Improvement

Safety

Informatics

Peer Review: _____   Faculty Review: _____

Grade Tracker

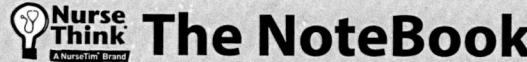
Related Concepts

Related Exemplars/Diseases

Reading/Resources - Clinical Judgment

Class/Lab/Clinical – Clinical Judgment

Priority Assessments or Cues

1

2

3

Priority Labs & Diagnostics

1

2

3

Priority Nursing Interventions

1

2

3

Priority Medications

1

2

3

Priority Potential & Actual Complications

1

2

3

Priority Collaborative Goals

1

2

3

NurseThink® Quick

Cushing Symptoms	Cushing Syndrome	
3 S's	***Cushing***	
Sugar (hyperglycemia)	**C**entral obesity	
Salt (hypernatremia)	**U**rinary free cortisol and glucose increase	
Sex (excess androgens)	**S**triate/Suppressed immunity	
	Hypercortisolism/Hypertension/ Hyperglycemia/ Hirsuism	
	Iatrogenic (Increased administration of corticosteroids)	
	Noniatrogenic (Neoplasms)	
	Glucose intolerance/ Growth retardation	

NEXT GEN LEARNING – NCLEX® TEST PLAN

Safe and Effective Care: Management of Care, Coordinated Care, Safety and Infection Control

Health Promotion and Maintenance

Psychosocial Integrity

Physiological Integrity: Basic Care and Comfort, Pharmacological and Parenteral Therapies, Reduction of Risk Potential, and Physiological Adaptation

QUALITY AND SAFETY COMPETENCIES

Patient-Centered Care

Teamwork and Collaboration

Evidence-Based Practice

Quality Improvement

Safety

Informatics

Peer Review: _____   Faculty Review: _____

Grade Tracker

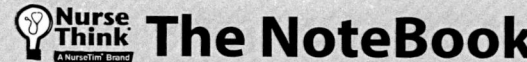
Related Concepts

Related Exemplars/Diseases

Reading/Resources - Clinical Judgment

Class/Lab/Clinical – Clinical Judgment

Priority Assessments or Cues

1

2

3

Priority Labs & Diagnostics

1

2

3

Priority Nursing Interventions

1

2

3

Priority Medications

1

2

3

Priority Potential & Actual Complications

1

2

3

Priority Collaborative Goals

1

2

3

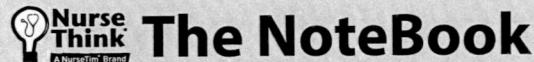
NurseThink® Quick

Crohn's Disease Symptoms		
Christmas		
Cobblestones		
High temperature		
Reduced lumen		
Intestinal fistulae		
Skip lesions		
Transmural		
Malabsorption		
Abdominal pain		
Submucosal fibrosis		

NEXT GEN LEARNING – NCLEX® TEST PLAN

Safe and Effective Care: Management of Care, Coordinated Care, Safety and Infection Control

Health Promotion and Maintenance

Psychosocial Integrity

Physiological Integrity: Basic Care and Comfort, Pharmacological and Parenteral Therapies, Reduction of Risk Potential, and Physiological Adaptation

QUALITY AND SAFETY COMPETENCIES

Patient-Centered Care

Teamwork and Collaboration

Evidence-Based Practice

Quality Improvement

Safety

Informatics

Peer Review: _____   Faculty Review: _____

Grade Tracker

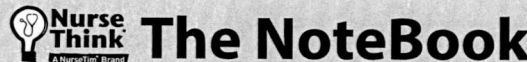

Related Concepts	Related Exemplars/Diseases

Reading/Resources - Clinical Judgment	Class/Lab/Clinical – Clinical Judgment
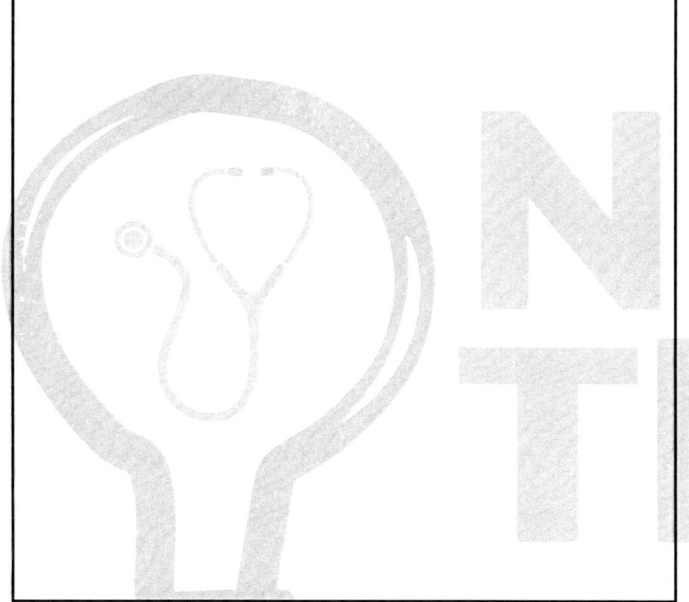	

Priority Assessments or Cues	Priority Labs & Diagnostics	Priority Nursing Interventions
1 2 3	1 2 3	1 2 3

Priority Medications	Priority Potential & Actual Complications	Priority Collaborative Goals
1 2 3	1 2 3	1 2 3

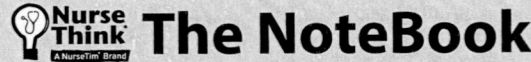

NurseThink® Quick

NEXT GEN LEARNING – NCLEX® TEST PLAN

Safe and Effective Care: Management of Care, Coordinated Care, Safety and Infection Control

Health Promotion and Maintenance

Psychosocial Integrity

Physiological Integrity: Basic Care and Comfort, Pharmacological and Parenteral Therapies, Reduction of Risk Potential, and Physiological Adaptation

QUALITY AND SAFETY COMPETENCIES

Patient-Centered Care

Teamwork and Collaboration

Evidence-Based Practice

Quality Improvement

Safety

Informatics

Peer Review: _____   Faculty Review: _____

Grade Tracker

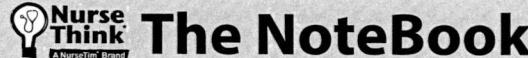
Related Concepts

Related Exemplars/Diseases

Reading/Resources - Clinical Judgment

Class/Lab/Clinical – Clinical Judgment

Priority Assessments or Cues
1
2
3

Priority Labs & Diagnostics
1
2
3

Priority Nursing Interventions
1
2
3

Priority Medications
1
2
3

Priority Potential & Actual Complications
1
2
3

Priority Collaborative Goals
1
2
3

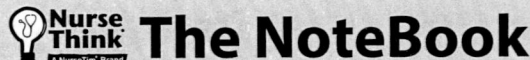
NurseThink® Quick

GI Obstruction: Symptoms	Small Bowel Obstruction: Causes	
PV D & C **P**ain **V**omiting **D**istension **C**onstipation	***Shavit*** **S**tone **H**ernia **A**dhesions **V**olvulus **I**ntussusception **T**umor	

NEXT GEN LEARNING – NCLEX® TEST PLAN

Safe and Effective Care: Management of Care, Coordinated Care, Safety and Infection Control

Health Promotion and Maintenance

Psychosocial Integrity

Physiological Integrity: Basic Care and Comfort, Pharmacological and Parenteral Therapies, Reduction of Risk Potential, and Physiological Adaptation

QUALITY AND SAFETY COMPETENCIES

Patient-Centered Care

Teamwork and Collaboration

Evidence-Based Practice

Quality Improvement

Safety

Informatics

Peer Review: _____   Faculty Review: _____

Grade Tracker

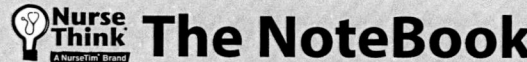
Related Concepts	Related Exemplars/Diseases

Reading/Resources - Clinical Judgment	Class/Lab/Clinical – Clinical Judgment

Priority Assessments or Cues

1

2

3

Priority Labs & Diagnostics

1

2

3

Priority Nursing Interventions

1

2

3

Priority Medications

1

2

3

Priority Potential & Actual Complications

1

2

3

Priority Collaborative Goals

1

2

3

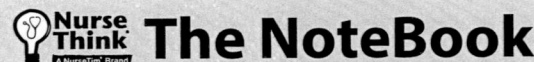
NurseThink® Quick

IBD: Surgery Indications		
I Chop		
Infection		
Carcinoma		
Hemorrhage		
Obstruction		
Perforation		

NEXT GEN LEARNING – NCLEX® TEST PLAN

Safe and Effective Care: Management of Care, Coordinated Care, Safety and Infection Control

Health Promotion and Maintenance

Psychosocial Integrity

Physiological Integrity: Basic Care and Comfort, Pharmacological and Parenteral Therapies, Reduction of Risk Potential, and Physiological Adaptation

QUALITY AND SAFETY COMPETENCIES

Patient-Centered Care

Teamwork and Collaboration

Evidence-Based Practice

Quality Improvement

Safety

Informatics

Peer Review: _____   Faculty Review: _____

Grade Tracker

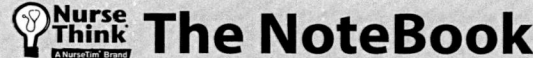
Related Concepts

Related Exemplars/Diseases

Reading/Resources - Clinical Judgment

Class/Lab/Clinical – Clinical Judgment

Priority Assessments or Cues

1

2

3

Priority Labs & Diagnostics

1

2

3

Priority Nursing Interventions

1

2

3

Priority Medications

1

2

3

Priority Potential & Actual Complications

1

2

3

Priority Collaborative Goals

1

2

3

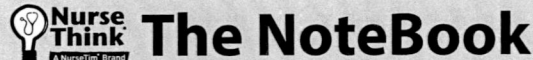
NurseThink® Quick

NEXT GEN LEARNING – NCLEX® TEST PLAN

Safe and Effective Care: Management of Care, Coordinated Care, Safety and Infection Control

Health Promotion and Maintenance

Psychosocial Integrity

Physiological Integrity: Basic Care and Comfort, Pharmacological and Parenteral Therapies, Reduction of Risk Potential, and Physiological Adaptation

QUALITY AND SAFETY COMPETENCIES

Patient-Centered Care

Teamwork and Collaboration

Evidence-Based Practice

Quality Improvement

Safety

Informatics

Peer Review: _____   Faculty Review: _____

Grade Tracker

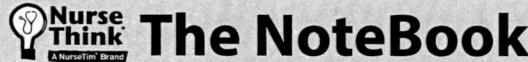
Related Concepts

Related Exemplars/Diseases

Reading/Resources - Clinical Judgment

Class/Lab/Clinical – Clinical Judgment

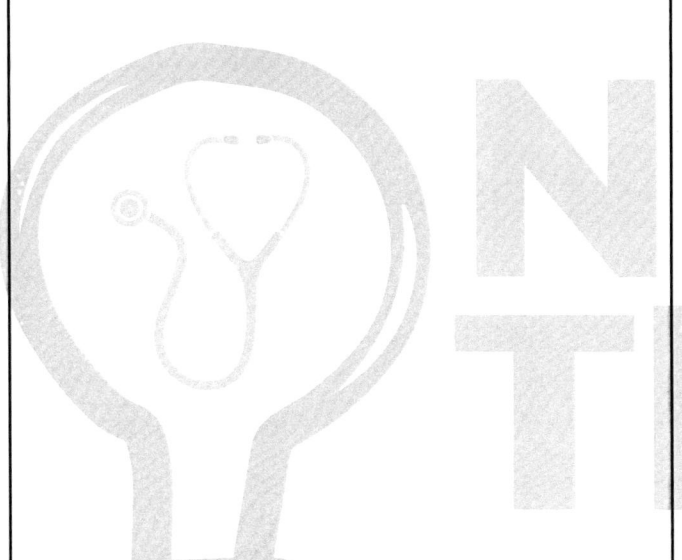

Priority Assessments or Cues

1

2

3

Priority Labs & Diagnostics

1

2

3

Priority Nursing Interventions

1

2

3

Priority Medications

1

2

3

Priority Potential & Actual Complications

1

2

3

Priority Collaborative Goals

1

2

3

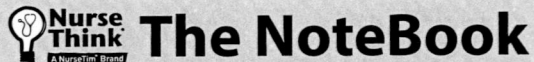
NurseThink® Quick

Ulcerative Colitis: Definition of a severe attack	**Ulcerative Colitis: Complications**	
A State	***Past Colitis***	
Anemia less than 10 g/dL	**P**yoderma gangrenosum	
Stool frequency greater than 6 stills/day with blood	**A**nkylosing spondylitis	
Temperature greater than 37.5	**S**clerosing pericholangities	
Albumin less than 30g/L	**T**oxic megacolon	
Tachycardia greater than 90bpm	**C**olon carcinoma	
ESR greater than 30 mm/hr		

NEXT GEN LEARNING – NCLEX® TEST PLAN

Safe and Effective Care: Management of Care, Coordinated Care, Safety and Infection Control

Health Promotion and Maintenance

Psychosocial Integrity

Physiological Integrity: Basic Care and Comfort, Pharmacological and Parenteral Therapies, Reduction of Risk Potential, and Physiological Adaptation

QUALITY AND SAFETY COMPETENCIES

Patient-Centered Care

Teamwork and Collaboration

Evidence-Based Practice

Quality Improvement

Safety

Informatics

Peer Review: _____ Faculty Review: _____

Grade Tracker

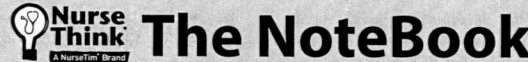

Related Concepts	**Related Exemplars/Diseases**

Reading/Resources - Clinical Judgment	**Class/Lab/Clinical – Clinical Judgment**

Priority Assessments or Cues	**Priority Labs & Diagnostics**	**Priority Nursing Interventions**
1	1	1
2	2	2
3	3	3

Priority Medications	**Priority Potential & Actual Complications**	**Priority Collaborative Goals**
1	1	1
2	2	2
3	3	3

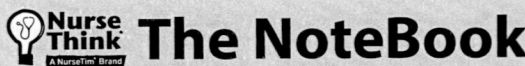
NurseThink® Quick

NEXT GEN LEARNING – NCLEX® TEST PLAN

Safe and Effective Care: Management of Care, Coordinated Care, Safety and Infection Control

Health Promotion and Maintenance

Psychosocial Integrity

Physiological Integrity: Basic Care and Comfort, Pharmacological and Parenteral Therapies, Reduction of Risk Potential, and Physiological Adaptation

QUALITY AND SAFETY COMPETENCIES

Patient-Centered Care

Teamwork and Collaboration

Evidence-Based Practice

Quality Improvement

Safety

Informatics

Peer Review: _____   Faculty Review: _____

Grade Tracker

Related Concepts

Related Exemplars/Diseases

Reading/Resources - Clinical Judgment

Class/Lab/Clinical – Clinical Judgment

Priority Assessments or Cues
1
2
3

Priority Labs & Diagnostics
1
2
3

Priority Nursing Interventions
1
2
3

Priority Medications
1

2

3

Priority Potential & Actual Complications
1

2

3

Priority Collaborative Goals
1

2

3

NurseThink® Quick

Hyperglycemia
(Skin) Hot and Dry: sugar's high
(Skin) Cold and Clammy: need some candy

Diabetes: Signs and Symptoms
3 P's
Polydipsia
Polyphagia
Polyuria

Diabetes Complications
Knives
Kidney
Neuropathy
Infection
Vascular
Eyes
Skin lesions

Diabetic Ketoacidosis: Treatment
Fire
Fluids
Insulin
Replace
Electrolytes

NEXT GEN LEARNING – NCLEX® TEST PLAN

Safe and Effective Care: Management of Care, Coordinated Care, Safety and Infection Control

Health Promotion and Maintenance

Psychosocial Integrity

Physiological Integrity: Basic Care and Comfort, Pharmacological and Parenteral Therapies, Reduction of Risk Potential, and Physiological Adaptation

QUALITY AND SAFETY COMPETENCIES

Patient-Centered Care

Teamwork and Collaboration

Evidence-Based Practice

Quality Improvement

Safety

Informatics

Peer Review: _____   Faculty Review: _____

Grade Tracker

Related Concepts

Related Exemplars/Diseases

Reading/Resources - Clinical Judgment

Class/Lab/Clinical – Clinical Judgment

Priority Assessments or Cues

1
2
3

Priority Labs & Diagnostics

1
2
3

Priority Nursing Interventions

1
2
3

Priority Medications

1
2
3

Priority Potential & Actual Complications

1
2
3

Priority Collaborative Goals

1
2
3

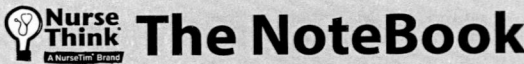
NurseThink® Quick

NEXT GEN LEARNING – NCLEX® TEST PLAN

Safe and Effective Care: Management of Care, Coordinated Care, Safety and Infection Control

Health Promotion and Maintenance

Psychosocial Integrity

Physiological Integrity: Basic Care and Comfort, Pharmacological and Parenteral Therapies, Reduction of Risk Potential, and Physiological Adaptation

QUALITY AND SAFETY COMPETENCIES

Patient-Centered Care

Teamwork and Collaboration

Evidence-Based Practice

Quality Improvement

Safety

Informatics

Peer Review: _____   Faculty Review: _____

Grade Tracker

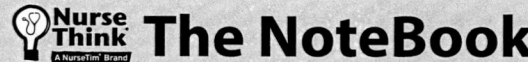

Related Concepts	**Related Exemplars/Diseases**

Reading/Resources - Clinical Judgment	**Class/Lab/Clinical – Clinical Judgment**

Priority Assessments or Cues	**Priority Labs & Diagnostics**	**Priority Nursing Interventions**
1	1	1
2	2	2
3	3	3

Priority Medications	**Priority Potential & Actual Complications**	**Priority Collaborative Goals**
1	1	1
2	2	2
3	3	3

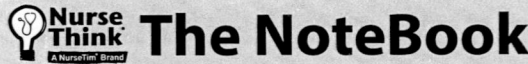
NurseThink® Quick

NEXT GEN LEARNING – NCLEX® TEST PLAN

Safe and Effective Care: Management of Care, Coordinated Care, Safety and Infection Control

Health Promotion and Maintenance

Psychosocial Integrity

Physiological Integrity: Basic Care and Comfort, Pharmacological and Parenteral Therapies, Reduction of Risk Potential, and Physiological Adaptation

QUALITY AND SAFETY COMPETENCIES

Patient-Centered Care

Teamwork and Collaboration

Evidence-Based Practice

Quality Improvement

Safety

Informatics

Peer Review: _____   Faculty Review: _____

Grade Tracker

Related Concepts	Related Exemplars/Diseases

Reading/Resources - Clinical Judgment	Class/Lab/Clinical – Clinical Judgment

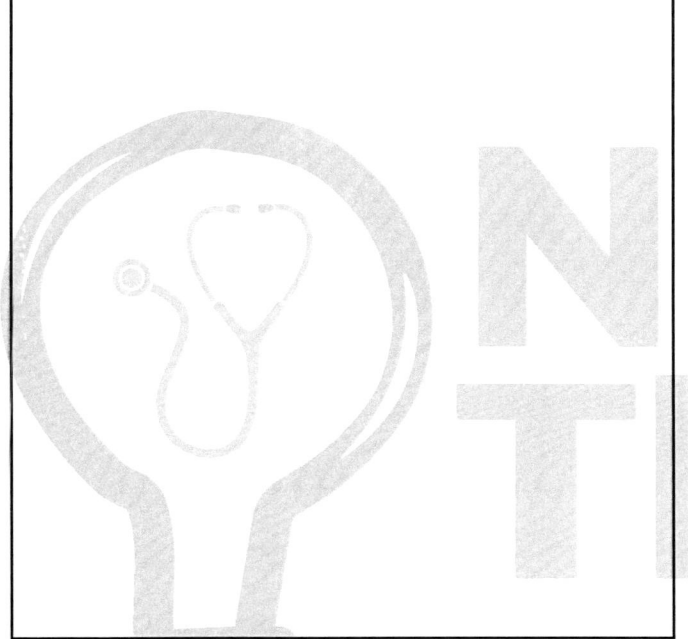

Priority Assessments or Cues
1
2
3

Priority Labs & Diagnostics
1
2
3

Priority Nursing Interventions
1
2
3

Priority Medications
1
2
3

Priority Potential & Actual Complications
1
2
3

Priority Collaborative Goals
1
2
3

NurseThink® Quick

NEXT GEN LEARNING – NCLEX® TEST PLAN

Safe and Effective Care: Management of Care, Coordinated Care, Safety and Infection Control

Health Promotion and Maintenance

Psychosocial Integrity

Physiological Integrity: Basic Care and Comfort, Pharmacological and Parenteral Therapies, Reduction of Risk Potential, and Physiological Adaptation

QUALITY AND SAFETY COMPETENCIES

Patient-Centered Care

Teamwork and Collaboration

Evidence-Based Practice

Quality Improvement

Safety

Informatics

Peer Review: _____   Faculty Review: _____

Grade Tracker

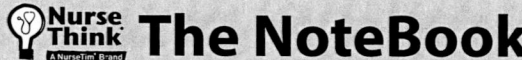
Related Concepts	**Related Exemplars/Diseases**

Reading/Resources - Clinical Judgment	**Class/Lab/Clinical – Clinical Judgment**

Priority Assessments or Cues

1

2

3

Priority Labs & Diagnostics

1

2

3

Priority Nursing Interventions

1

2

3

Priority Medications

1

2

3

Priority Potential & Actual Complications

1

2

3

Priority Collaborative Goals

1

2

3

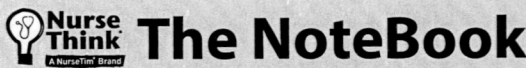
NurseThink® Quick

NEXT GEN LEARNING – NCLEX® TEST PLAN

Safe and Effective Care: Management of Care, Coordinated Care, Safety and Infection Control

Health Promotion and Maintenance

Psychosocial Integrity

Physiological Integrity: Basic Care and Comfort, Pharmacological and Parenteral Therapies, Reduction of Risk Potential, and Physiological Adaptation

QUALITY AND SAFETY COMPETENCIES

Patient-Centered Care

Teamwork and Collaboration

Evidence-Based Practice

Quality Improvement

Safety

Informatics

Peer Review: _____   Faculty Review: _____

Grade Tracker

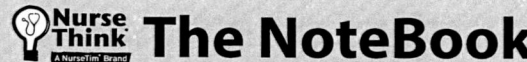
Related Concepts

Related Exemplars/Diseases

Reading/Resources - Clinical Judgment

Class/Lab/Clinical – Clinical Judgment

Priority Assessments or Cues

1

2

3

Priority Labs & Diagnostics

1

2

3

Priority Nursing Interventions

1

2

3

Priority Medications

1

2

3

Priority Potential & Actual Complications

1

2

3

Priority Collaborative Goals

1

2

3

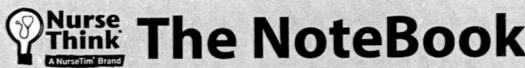
NurseThink® Quick

NEXT GEN LEARNING – NCLEX® TEST PLAN

Safe and Effective Care: Management of Care, Coordinated Care, Safety and Infection Control

Health Promotion and Maintenance

Psychosocial Integrity

Physiological Integrity: Basic Care and Comfort, Pharmacological and Parenteral Therapies, Reduction of Risk Potential, and Physiological Adaptation

QUALITY AND SAFETY COMPETENCIES

Patient-Centered Care

Teamwork and Collaboration

Evidence-Based Practice

Quality Improvement

Safety

Informatics

Peer Review: _____   Faculty Review: _____

Grade Tracker

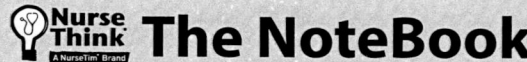
Related Concepts	Related Exemplars/Diseases

Reading/Resources - Clinical Judgment	Class/Lab/Clinical – Clinical Judgment

Priority Assessments or Cues	Priority Labs & Diagnostics	Priority Nursing Interventions
1	1	1
2	2	2
3	3	3

Priority Medications	Priority Potential & Actual Complications	Priority Collaborative Goals
1	1	1
2	2	2
3	3	3

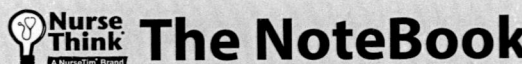
NurseThink® Quick

NEXT GEN LEARNING – NCLEX® TEST PLAN

Safe and Effective Care: Management of Care, Coordinated Care, Safety and Infection Control

Health Promotion and Maintenance

Psychosocial Integrity

Physiological Integrity: Basic Care and Comfort, Pharmacological and Parenteral Therapies, Reduction of Risk Potential, and Physiological Adaptation

QUALITY AND SAFETY COMPETENCIES

Patient-Centered Care

Teamwork and Collaboration

Evidence-Based Practice

Quality Improvement

Safety

Informatics

Peer Review: _____   Faculty Review: _____

Grade Tracker

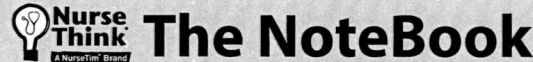
Related Concepts	**Related Exemplars/Diseases**

Reading/Resources - Clinical Judgment	**Class/Lab/Clinical – Clinical Judgment**

Priority Assessments or Cues	**Priority Labs & Diagnostics**	**Priority Nursing Interventions**
1	1	1
2	2	2
3	3	3

Priority Medications	**Priority Potential & Actual Complications**	**Priority Collaborative Goals**
1	1	1
2	2	2
3	3	3

NurseThink® Quick

SIADH: Inducing Drugs	SIADH: Causes	
ABCD	**SIADH**	
Analgesics: opioids, NSAIDs	**S**urgery	
Barbiturates	**I**ntracranial: infection, head injury, CVA	
Cyclophosphamide/Chlorpromazine/ Carbamazepine	**A**lveolar: cancer, pus	
Diuretic (thiazide)	**D**rugs	
	Hormonal: hypothyroid, low corticosteroid level	

NEXT GEN LEARNING – NCLEX® TEST PLAN

Safe and Effective Care: Management of Care, Coordinated Care, Safety and Infection Control

Health Promotion and Maintenance

Psychosocial Integrity

Physiological Integrity: Basic Care and Comfort, Pharmacological and Parenteral Therapies, Reduction of Risk Potential, and Physiological Adaptation

QUALITY AND SAFETY COMPETENCIES

Patient-Centered Care

Teamwork and Collaboration

Evidence-Based Practice

Quality Improvement

Safety

Informatics

Peer Review: _____   Faculty Review: _____

Grade Tracker

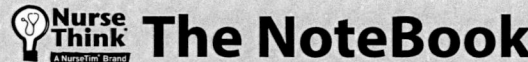
Related Concepts

Related Exemplars/Diseases

Reading/Resources - Clinical Judgment

Class/Lab/Clinical – Clinical Judgment

Priority Assessments or Cues

1

2

3

Priority Labs & Diagnostics

1

2

3

Priority Nursing Interventions

1

2

3

Priority Medications

1

2

3

Priority Potential & Actual Complications

1

2

3

Priority Collaborative Goals

1

2

3

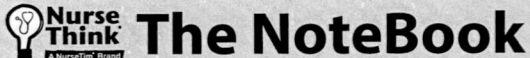
NurseThink® Quick

Thyroid Storm: Initial Management	Hyperthyroidism: Signs and Symptoms
PCP's **P**TU – 1gm PO **C**orticosteroids **P**ropranolol **S**SKI	**Thyroidism** **T**remor **H**eart rate up **Y**awning (fatigability) **R**estlessness **O**ligomenorrhea & amenorrhea **I**ntolerance to heat **D**iarrhea **I**rritability **S**weating **M**uscle wasting & weight loss

NEXT GEN LEARNING – NCLEX® TEST PLAN

Safe and Effective Care: Management of Care, Coordinated Care, Safety and Infection Control

Health Promotion and Maintenance

Psychosocial Integrity

Physiological Integrity: Basic Care and Comfort, Pharmacological and Parenteral Therapies, Reduction of Risk Potential, and Physiological Adaptation

QUALITY AND SAFETY COMPETENCIES

Patient-Centered Care

Teamwork and Collaboration

Evidence-Based Practice

Quality Improvement

Safety

Informatics

Peer Review: _____   Faculty Review: _____

Grade Tracker

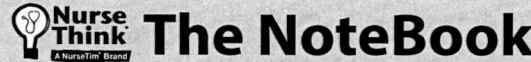
Related Concepts	Related Exemplars/Diseases

Reading/Resources - Clinical Judgment	Class/Lab/Clinical – Clinical Judgment
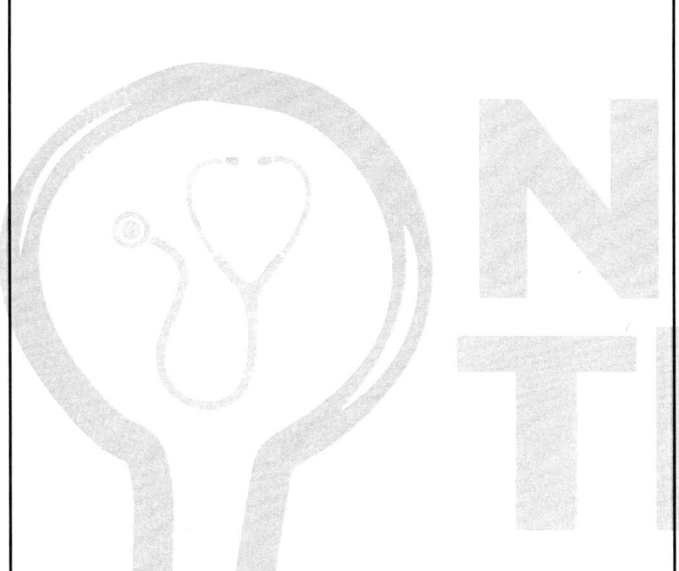	

Priority Assessments or Cues	Priority Labs & Diagnostics	Priority Nursing Interventions
1	1	1
2	2	2
3	3	3

Priority Medications	Priority Potential & Actual Complications	Priority Collaborative Goals
1	1	1
2	2	2
3	3	3

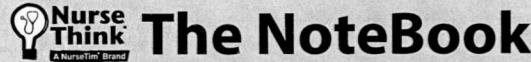
NurseThink® Quick

NEXT GEN LEARNING – NCLEX® TEST PLAN

Safe and Effective Care: Management of Care, Coordinated Care, Safety and Infection Control

Health Promotion and Maintenance

Psychosocial Integrity

Physiological Integrity: Basic Care and Comfort, Pharmacological and Parenteral Therapies, Reduction of Risk Potential, and Physiological Adaptation

QUALITY AND SAFETY COMPETENCIES

Patient-Centered Care

Teamwork and Collaboration

Evidence-Based Practice

Quality Improvement

Safety

Informatics

Peer Review: _____   Faculty Review: _____

Grade Tracker

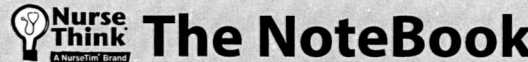
Related Concepts	**Related Exemplars/Diseases**

Reading/Resources - Clinical Judgment	**Class/Lab/Clinical – Clinical Judgment**

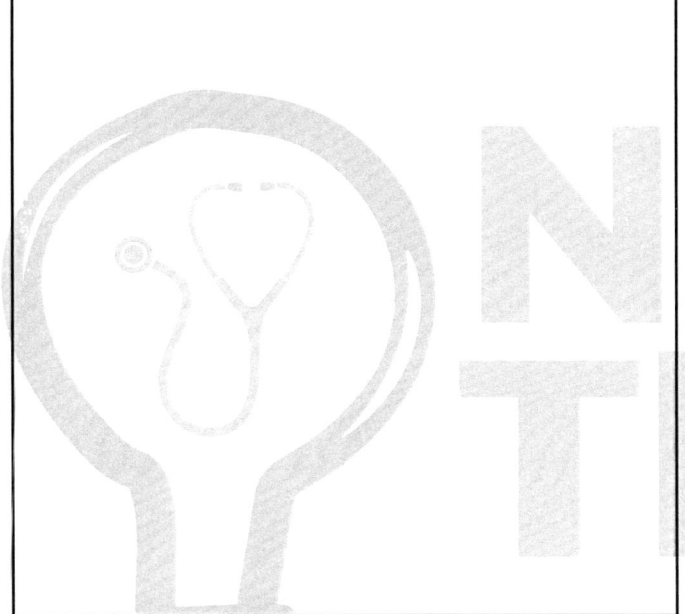

Priority Assessments or Cues	**Priority Labs & Diagnostics**	**Priority Nursing Interventions**
1	1	1
2	2	2
3	3	3

Priority Medications	**Priority Potential & Actual Complications**	**Priority Collaborative Goals**
1	1	1
2	2	2
3	3	3

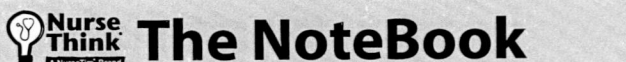
NurseThink® Quick

NEXT GEN LEARNING – NCLEX® TEST PLAN

Safe and Effective Care: Management of Care, Coordinated Care, Safety and Infection Control

Health Promotion and Maintenance

Psychosocial Integrity

Physiological Integrity: Basic Care and Comfort, Pharmacological and Parenteral Therapies, Reduction of Risk Potential, and Physiological Adaptation

QUALITY AND SAFETY COMPETENCIES

Patient-Centered Care

Teamwork and Collaboration

Evidence-Based Practice

Quality Improvement

Safety

Informatics

Peer Review: _____   Faculty Review: _____

Grade Tracker

Related Concepts

Related Exemplars/Diseases

Reading/Resources - Clinical Judgment

Class/Lab/Clinical – Clinical Judgment

Priority Assessments or Cues

1
2
3

Priority Labs & Diagnostics

1
2
3

Priority Nursing Interventions

1
2
3

Priority Medications

1
2
3

Priority Potential & Actual Complications

1
2
3

Priority Collaborative Goals

1
2
3

NurseThink® Quick

H. Pylori Treatment	**Peptic Ulcer: Associated Causes**	
Please Make Tummy Better	*Shazam*	
Proton pump inhibitor	**S**moking	
Metronidazole	**H**ypercalcemia	
Tetracycline	**A**spirin	
Bismuth	**Z**ollinger-Ellison	
	Acidity	
	MEN Type 1	

NEXT GEN LEARNING – NCLEX® TEST PLAN

Safe and Effective Care: Management of Care, Coordinated Care, Safety and Infection Control

Health Promotion and Maintenance

Psychosocial Integrity

Physiological Integrity: Basic Care and Comfort, Pharmacological and Parenteral Therapies, Reduction of Risk Potential, and Physiological Adaptation

QUALITY AND SAFETY COMPETENCIES

Patient-Centered Care

Teamwork and Collaboration

Evidence-Based Practice

Quality Improvement

Safety

Informatics

Peer Review: _____   Faculty Review: _____

Grade Tracker

Related Concepts	Related Exemplars/Diseases

Reading/Resources - Clinical Judgment	Class/Lab/Clinical – Clinical Judgment

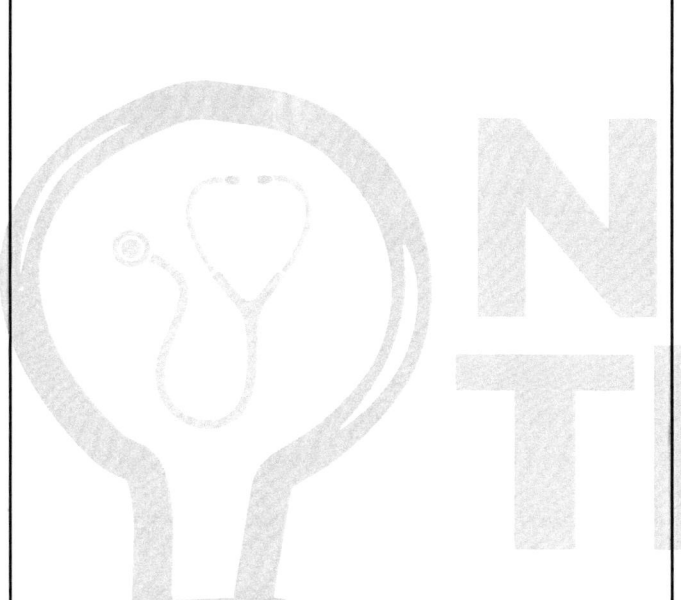

Priority Assessments or Cues	Priority Labs & Diagnostics	Priority Nursing Interventions
1	1	1
2	2	2
3	3	3

Priority Medications	Priority Potential & Actual Complications	Priority Collaborative Goals
1	1	1
2	2	2
3	3	3

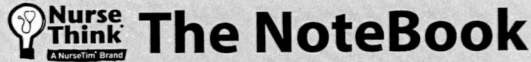
NurseThink® Quick

NEXT GEN LEARNING – NCLEX® TEST PLAN

Safe and Effective Care: Management of Care, Coordinated Care, Safety and Infection Control

Health Promotion and Maintenance

Psychosocial Integrity

Physiological Integrity: Basic Care and Comfort, Pharmacological and Parenteral Therapies, Reduction of Risk Potential, and Physiological Adaptation

QUALITY AND SAFETY COMPETENCIES

Patient-Centered Care

Teamwork and Collaboration

Evidence-Based Practice

Quality Improvement

Safety

Informatics

Peer Review: _____   Faculty Review: _____

Grade Tracker

Related Concepts	**Related Exemplars/Diseases**

Reading/Resources - Clinical Judgment	**Class/Lab/Clinical – Clinical Judgment**
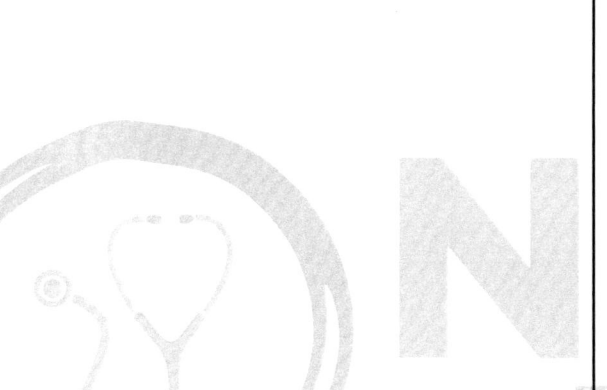	

Priority Assessments or Cues	**Priority Labs & Diagnostics**	**Priority Nursing Interventions**
1	1	1
2	2	2
3	3	3

Priority Medications	**Priority Potential & Actual Complications**	**Priority Collaborative Goals**
1	1	1
2	2	2
3	3	3

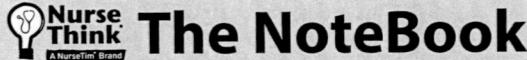
NurseThink® Quick

Renal Failure: Management		
AEIOU **A**nemia/Acidosis **E**lectrolytes and fluids **I**nfections **O**ther measures (nutrition, nausea, vomiting) **U**remia		

NEXT GEN LEARNING – NCLEX® TEST PLAN

Safe and Effective Care: Management of Care, Coordinated Care, Safety and Infection Control

Health Promotion and Maintenance

Psychosocial Integrity

Physiological Integrity: Basic Care and Comfort, Pharmacological and Parenteral Therapies, Reduction of Risk Potential, and Physiological Adaptation

QUALITY AND SAFETY COMPETENCIES

Patient-Centered Care

Teamwork and Collaboration

Evidence-Based Practice

Quality Improvement

Safety

Informatics

Peer Review: _____   Faculty Review: _____

Grade Tracker

Related Concepts

Related Exemplars/Diseases

Reading/Resources - Clinical Judgment

Class/Lab/Clinical – Clinical Judgment

Priority Assessments or Cues

1

2

3

Priority Labs & Diagnostics

1

2

3

Priority Nursing Interventions

1

2

3

Priority Medications

1

2

3

Priority Potential & Actual Complications

1

2

3

Priority Collaborative Goals

1

2

3

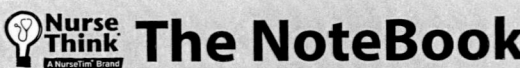
NurseThink® Quick

NEXT GEN LEARNING – NCLEX® TEST PLAN

Safe and Effective Care: Management of Care, Coordinated Care, Safety and Infection Control

Health Promotion and Maintenance

Psychosocial Integrity

Physiological Integrity: Basic Care and Comfort, Pharmacological and Parenteral Therapies, Reduction of Risk Potential, and Physiological Adaptation

QUALITY AND SAFETY COMPETENCIES

Patient-Centered Care

Teamwork and Collaboration

Evidence-Based Practice

Quality Improvement

Safety

Informatics

Peer Review: _____   Faculty Review: _____

Grade Tracker

Related Concepts

Related Exemplars/Diseases

Reading/Resources - Clinical Judgment

Class/Lab/Clinical – Clinical Judgment

Priority Assessments or Cues

1

2

3

Priority Labs & Diagnostics

1

2

3

Priority Nursing Interventions

1

2

3

Priority Medications

1

2

3

Priority Potential & Actual Complications

1

2

3

Priority Collaborative Goals

1

2

3

NurseThink® Quick

Chronic Renal Failure: Causes	**Renal Failure: Symptoms/Signs**	**Renal Failure: Consequences**
Glad Shop	*Get Vinny Prepared, He's Not Making Big Pee*	*ABCDEFG*
Glomerulonephritis	**G**I motility	**A**nemia
Lupus	**V**omiting	**B**one alterations
Analgesics	**P**ruritus	**C**ardiopulmonary
Diabetes	**H**eadache	**V**itamin D loss
Systemic vascular disease	**N**ausea	**E**lectrolyte imbalance
Hypertension	**M**alaise	**F**everous infections
Obstruction	**B**reathlessness	**G**I disturbances
Polycystic kidney disease	**P**igmentation	

NEXT GEN LEARNING – NCLEX® TEST PLAN

Safe and Effective Care: Management of Care, Coordinated Care, Safety and Infection Control

Health Promotion and Maintenance

Psychosocial Integrity

Physiological Integrity: Basic Care and Comfort, Pharmacological and Parenteral Therapies, Reduction of Risk Potential, and Physiological Adaptation

QUALITY AND SAFETY COMPETENCIES

Patient-Centered Care

Teamwork and Collaboration

Evidence-Based Practice

Quality Improvement

Safety

Informatics

Peer Review: _____   Faculty Review: _____

Grade Tracker

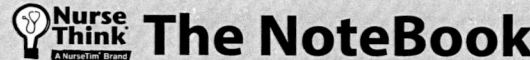
Related Concepts

Related Exemplars/Diseases

Reading/Resources - Clinical Judgment

Class/Lab/Clinical – Clinical Judgment

Priority Assessments or Cues

1

2

3

Priority Labs & Diagnostics

1

2

3

Priority Nursing Interventions

1

2

3

Priority Medications

1

2

3

Priority Potential & Actual Complications

1

2

3

Priority Collaborative Goals

1

2

3

NurseThink® Quick

NEXT GEN LEARNING – NCLEX® TEST PLAN

Safe and Effective Care: Management of Care, Coordinated Care, Safety and Infection Control

Health Promotion and Maintenance

Psychosocial Integrity

Physiological Integrity: Basic Care and Comfort, Pharmacological and Parenteral Therapies, Reduction of Risk Potential, and Physiological Adaptation

QUALITY AND SAFETY COMPETENCIES

Patient-Centered Care

Teamwork and Collaboration

Evidence-Based Practice

Quality Improvement

Safety

Informatics

Peer Review: _____ Faculty Review: _____

Grade Tracker

Related Concepts

Related Exemplars/Diseases

Reading/Resources - Clinical Judgment

Class/Lab/Clinical – Clinical Judgment

Priority Assessments or Cues

1

2

3

Priority Labs & Diagnostics

1

2

3

Priority Nursing Interventions

1

2

3

Priority Medications

1

2

3

Priority Potential & Actual Complications

1

2

3

Priority Collaborative Goals

1

2

3

NurseThink® Quick

NEXT GEN LEARNING – NCLEX® TEST PLAN

Safe and Effective Care: Management of Care, Coordinated Care, Safety and Infection Control

Health Promotion and Maintenance

Psychosocial Integrity

Physiological Integrity: Basic Care and Comfort, Pharmacological and Parenteral Therapies, Reduction of Risk Potential, and Physiological Adaptation

QUALITY AND SAFETY COMPETENCIES

Patient-Centered Care

Teamwork and Collaboration

Evidence-Based Practice

Quality Improvement

Safety

Informatics

Peer Review: _____   Faculty Review: _____

Grade Tracker

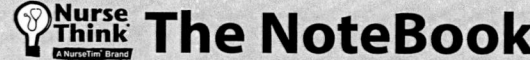
Related Concepts	Related Exemplars/Diseases

Reading/Resources - Clinical Judgment	Class/Lab/Clinical – Clinical Judgment

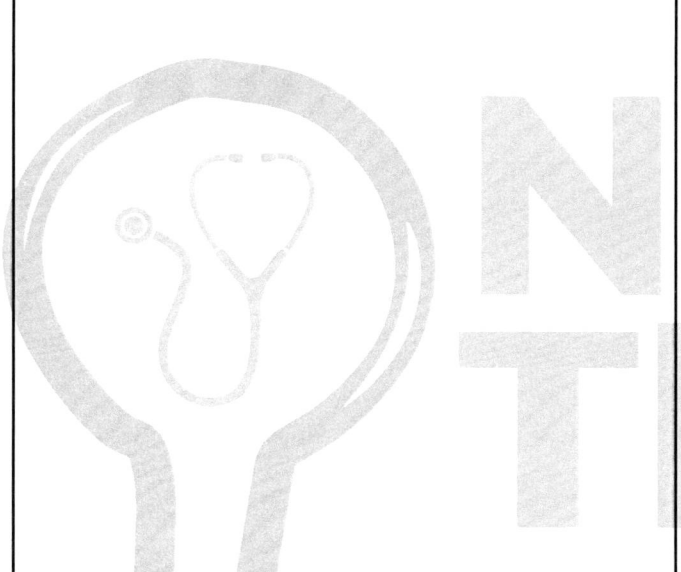

Priority Assessments or Cues	Priority Labs & Diagnostics	Priority Nursing Interventions
1	1	1
2	2	2
3	3	3

Priority Medications	Priority Potential & Actual Complications	Priority Collaborative Goals
1	1	1
2	2	2
3	3	3

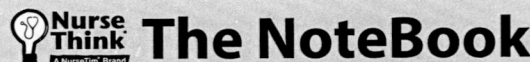
NurseThink® Quick

Asthma: Precipitating Factors ***Diplomat*** **D**rugs (aspirin, NSAIDs, Beta blockers) **I**nfections **P**ollutants (home, work) **L**aughter (emotion) **O** – Esophageal Reflux (nocturnal asthma) **M**ites **A**ctivity and Exercise **T**emperature (cold)	**Asthma: Treatments** ***Asthma*** **A**drenergics **S**teroids **T**heophyllines **H**ydration **M**ask O2 **A**BGs	

NEXT GEN LEARNING – NCLEX® TEST PLAN

Safe and Effective Care: Management of Care, Coordinated Care, Safety and Infection Control

Health Promotion and Maintenance

Psychosocial Integrity

Physiological Integrity: Basic Care and Comfort, Pharmacological and Parenteral Therapies, Reduction of Risk Potential, and Physiological Adaptation

QUALITY AND SAFETY COMPETENCIES

Patient-Centered Care

Teamwork and Collaboration

Evidence-Based Practice

Quality Improvement

Safety

Informatics

Peer Review: _____   Faculty Review: _____

Grade Tracker

Related Concepts

Related Exemplars/Diseases

Reading/Resources - Clinical Judgment

Class/Lab/Clinical – Clinical Judgment

Priority Assessments or Cues

1
2
3

Priority Labs & Diagnostics

1
2
3

Priority Nursing Interventions

1
2
3

Priority Medications

1
2
3

Priority Potential & Actual Complications

1
2
3

Priority Collaborative Goals

1
2
3

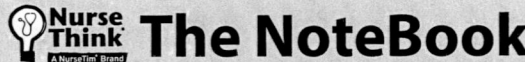
NurseThink® Quick

COPD:	COPD: 4 Types	Emphysema
Emphysema has the letter P = Pink puffer	***ABCDE***	***Cigarettes Is Primary Problem***
Bronchitis has the letter B = Blue bloater	**A**sthma	**C**igarettes
	Bronchiectasis	**I**nflammation healed to scar
	Chronic bronchitis	**P**rotease inhibitor deficiency
	Dyspnea	**P**neumothorax
	Emphysema	

NEXT GEN LEARNING – NCLEX® TEST PLAN

Safe and Effective Care: Management of Care, Coordinated Care, Safety and Infection Control

Health Promotion and Maintenance

Psychosocial Integrity

Physiological Integrity: Basic Care and Comfort, Pharmacological and Parenteral Therapies, Reduction of Risk Potential, and Physiological Adaptation

QUALITY AND SAFETY COMPETENCIES

Patient-Centered Care

Teamwork and Collaboration

Evidence-Based Practice

Quality Improvement

Safety

Informatics

Peer Review: _____   Faculty Review: _____

Grade Tracker

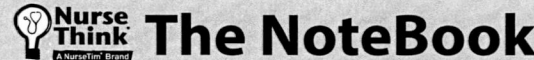
Related Concepts	Related Exemplars/Diseases

Reading/Resources - Clinical Judgment	Class/Lab/Clinical – Clinical Judgment
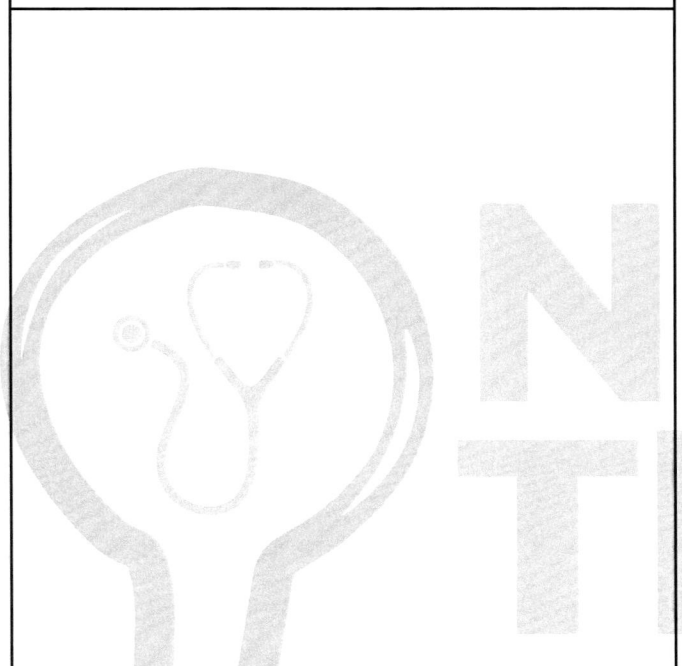	

Priority Assessments or Cues	Priority Labs & Diagnostics	Priority Nursing Interventions
1	1	1
2	2	2
3	3	3

Priority Medications	Priority Potential & Actual Complications	Priority Collaborative Goals
1	1	1
2	2	2
3	3	3

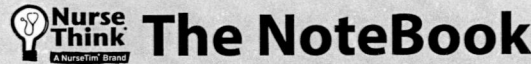
NurseThink® Quick

NEXT GEN LEARNING – NCLEX® TEST PLAN

Safe and Effective Care: Management of Care, Coordinated Care, Safety and Infection Control

Health Promotion and Maintenance

Psychosocial Integrity

Physiological Integrity: Basic Care and Comfort, Pharmacological and Parenteral Therapies, Reduction of Risk Potential, and Physiological Adaptation

QUALITY AND SAFETY COMPETENCIES

Patient-Centered Care

Teamwork and Collaboration

Evidence-Based Practice

Quality Improvement

Safety

Informatics

Peer Review: _____   Faculty Review: _____

Grade Tracker

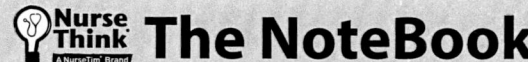
Related Concepts	**Related Exemplars/Diseases**

Reading/Resources - Clinical Judgment	**Class/Lab/Clinical – Clinical Judgment**

Priority Assessments or Cues	**Priority Labs & Diagnostics**	**Priority Nursing Interventions**
1	1	1
2	2	2
3	3	3

Priority Medications	**Priority Potential & Actual Complications**	**Priority Collaborative Goals**
1	1	1
2	2	2
3	3	3

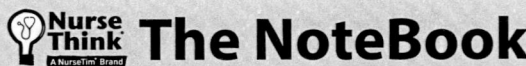
NurseThink® Quick

NEXT GEN LEARNING – NCLEX® TEST PLAN

Safe and Effective Care: Management of Care, Coordinated Care, Safety and Infection Control

Health Promotion and Maintenance

Psychosocial Integrity

Physiological Integrity: Basic Care and Comfort, Pharmacological and Parenteral Therapies, Reduction of Risk Potential, and Physiological Adaptation

QUALITY AND SAFETY COMPETENCIES

Patient-Centered Care

Teamwork and Collaboration

Evidence-Based Practice

Quality Improvement

Safety

Informatics

Peer Review: _____   Faculty Review: _____

Grade Tracker

Related Concepts

Related Exemplars/Diseases

Reading/Resources - Clinical Judgment

Class/Lab/Clinical – Clinical Judgment

Priority Assessments or Cues

1

2

3

Priority Labs & Diagnostics

1

2

3

Priority Nursing Interventions

1

2

3

Priority Medications

1

2

3

Priority Potential & Actual Complications

1

2

3

Priority Collaborative Goals

1

2

3

NurseThink® Quick

Acute Respiratory Failure: Type II (Hypoventilation) Criteria
50/50 Rule
PaCO2 >50
PaO2 <50 (on >50% oxygen)

Respiratory Depression Drugs
Stop
Sedatives and hypnotics
Trimethoprim
Opiates
Polymyxins

Ventilator Settings: Difference between A/C and SIMV Ventilation
A/C - Always assists (patient effort triggers vent breath delivery!)
SIMV - Sometimes assists

ARDS Causes
AAAARDDDDDSSS
Aspiration
Acute pancreatitis
Air embolism
Amniotic embolism
Radiation
DIC
Drugs
Dialysis
Drowning
Diffuse lung infection
Shock
Sepsis
Smoke inhalation

NEXT GEN LEARNING – NCLEX® TEST PLAN

Safe and Effective Care: Management of Care, Coordinated Care, Safety and Infection Control

Health Promotion and Maintenance

Psychosocial Integrity

Physiological Integrity: Basic Care and Comfort, Pharmacological and Parenteral Therapies, Reduction of Risk Potential, and Physiological Adaptation

QUALITY AND SAFETY COMPETENCIES

Patient-Centered Care

Teamwork and Collaboration

Evidence-Based Practice

Quality Improvement

Safety

Informatics

Peer Review: _____   Faculty Review: _____

Grade Tracker

Related Concepts

Related Exemplars/Diseases

Reading/Resources - Clinical Judgment

Class/Lab/Clinical – Clinical Judgment

Priority Assessments or Cues

1

2

3

Priority Labs & Diagnostics

1

2

3

Priority Nursing Interventions

1

2

3

Priority Medications

1

2

3

Priority Potential & Actual Complications

1

2

3

Priority Collaborative Goals

1

2

3

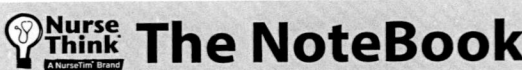
NurseThink® Quick

NEXT GEN LEARNING – NCLEX® TEST PLAN

Safe and Effective Care: Management of Care, Coordinated Care, Safety and Infection Control

Health Promotion and Maintenance

Psychosocial Integrity

Physiological Integrity: Basic Care and Comfort, Pharmacological and Parenteral Therapies, Reduction of Risk Potential, and Physiological Adaptation

QUALITY AND SAFETY COMPETENCIES

Patient-Centered Care

Teamwork and Collaboration

Evidence-Based Practice

Quality Improvement

Safety

Informatics

Peer Review: _____   Faculty Review: _____

Grade Tracker

Related Concepts

Related Exemplars/Diseases

Reading/Resources - Clinical Judgment

Class/Lab/Clinical – Clinical Judgment

Priority Assessments or Cues

1
2
3

Priority Labs & Diagnostics

1
2
3

Priority Nursing Interventions

1
2
3

Priority Medications

1

2

3

Priority Potential & Actual Complications

1

2

3

Priority Collaborative Goals

1

2

3

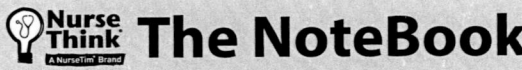
NurseThink® Quick

<table>
<tr><td></td><td></td><td></td></tr>
</table>

NEXT GEN LEARNING – NCLEX® TEST PLAN

Safe and Effective Care: Management of Care, Coordinated Care, Safety and Infection Control

Health Promotion and Maintenance

Psychosocial Integrity

Physiological Integrity: Basic Care and Comfort, Pharmacological and Parenteral Therapies, Reduction of Risk Potential, and Physiological Adaptation

QUALITY AND SAFETY COMPETENCIES

Patient-Centered Care

Teamwork and Collaboration

Evidence-Based Practice

Quality Improvement

Safety

Informatics

Peer Review: _____   Faculty Review: _____

Grade Tracker

<table>
<tr><td></td><td></td><td></td><td></td><td></td><td></td><td></td><td></td><td></td><td></td><td></td><td></td><td></td><td></td><td></td></tr>
</table>

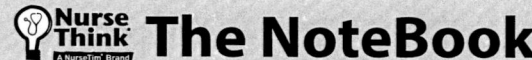

Related Concepts	Related Exemplars/Diseases

Reading/Resources - Clinical Judgment	Class/Lab/Clinical – Clinical Judgment

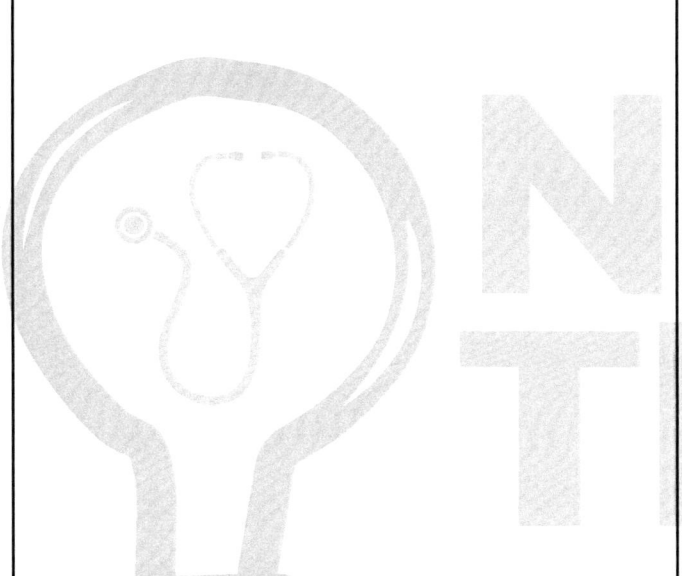

Priority Assessments or Cues	Priority Labs & Diagnostics	Priority Nursing Interventions
1	1	1
2	2	2
3	3	3

Priority Medications	Priority Potential & Actual Complications	Priority Collaborative Goals
1	1	1
2	2	2
3	3	3

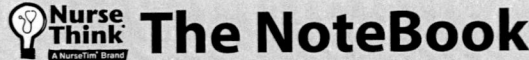

NurseThink® Quick

NEXT GEN LEARNING – NCLEX® TEST PLAN

Safe and Effective Care: Management of Care, Coordinated Care, Safety and Infection Control

Health Promotion and Maintenance

Psychosocial Integrity

Physiological Integrity: Basic Care and Comfort, Pharmacological and Parenteral Therapies, Reduction of Risk Potential, and Physiological Adaptation

QUALITY AND SAFETY COMPETENCIES

Patient-Centered Care

Teamwork and Collaboration

Evidence-Based Practice

Quality Improvement

Safety

Informatics

Peer Review: _____   Faculty Review: _____

Grade Tracker

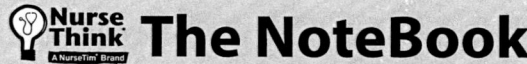
Related Concepts	**Related Exemplars/Diseases**

Reading/Resources - Clinical Judgment	**Class/Lab/Clinical – Clinical Judgment**

Priority Assessments or Cues	**Priority Labs & Diagnostics**	**Priority Nursing Interventions**
1	1	1
2	2	2
3	3	3

Priority Medications	**Priority Potential & Actual Complications**	**Priority Collaborative Goals**
1	1	1
2	2	2
3	3	3

NurseThink® Quick

NEXT GEN LEARNING – NCLEX® TEST PLAN

Safe and Effective Care: Management of Care, Coordinated Care, Safety and Infection Control

Health Promotion and Maintenance

Psychosocial Integrity

Physiological Integrity: Basic Care and Comfort, Pharmacological and Parenteral Therapies, Reduction of Risk Potential, and Physiological Adaptation

QUALITY AND SAFETY COMPETENCIES

Patient-Centered Care

Teamwork and Collaboration

Evidence-Based Practice

Quality Improvement

Safety

Informatics

Peer Review: _____   Faculty Review: _____

Grade Tracker

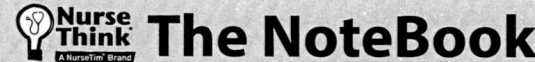
Related Concepts	Related Exemplars/Diseases

Reading/Resources - Clinical Judgment	Class/Lab/Clinical – Clinical Judgment
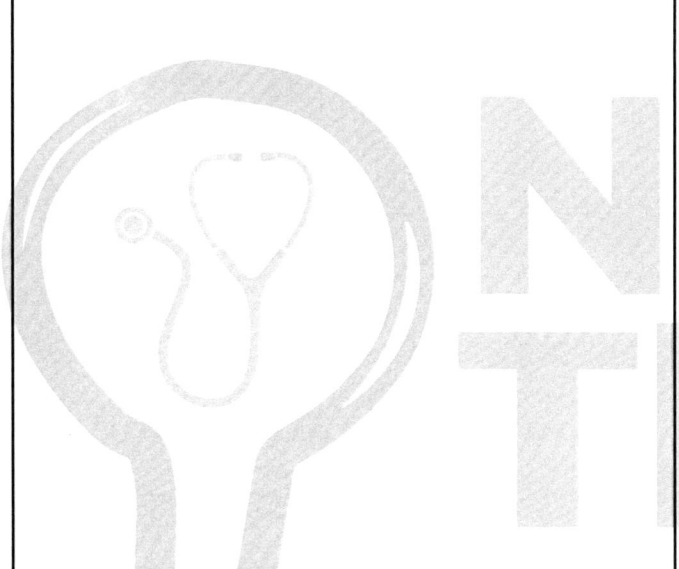	

Priority Assessments or Cues	Priority Labs & Diagnostics	Priority Nursing Interventions
1	1	1
2	2	2
3	3	3

Priority Medications	Priority Potential & Actual Complications	Priority Collaborative Goals
1	1	1
2	2	2
3	3	3

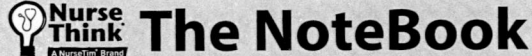
NurseThink® Quick

NEXT GEN LEARNING – NCLEX® TEST PLAN

Safe and Effective Care: Management of Care, Coordinated Care, Safety and Infection Control

Health Promotion and Maintenance

Psychosocial Integrity

Physiological Integrity: Basic Care and Comfort, Pharmacological and Parenteral Therapies, Reduction of Risk Potential, and Physiological Adaptation

QUALITY AND SAFETY COMPETENCIES

Patient-Centered Care

Teamwork and Collaboration

Evidence-Based Practice

Quality Improvement

Safety

Informatics

Peer Review: _____   Faculty Review: _____

Grade Tracker

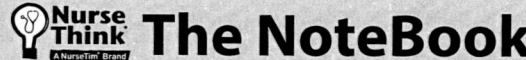

Related Concepts

Related Exemplars/Diseases

Reading/Resources - Clinical Judgment

Class/Lab/Clinical – Clinical Judgment

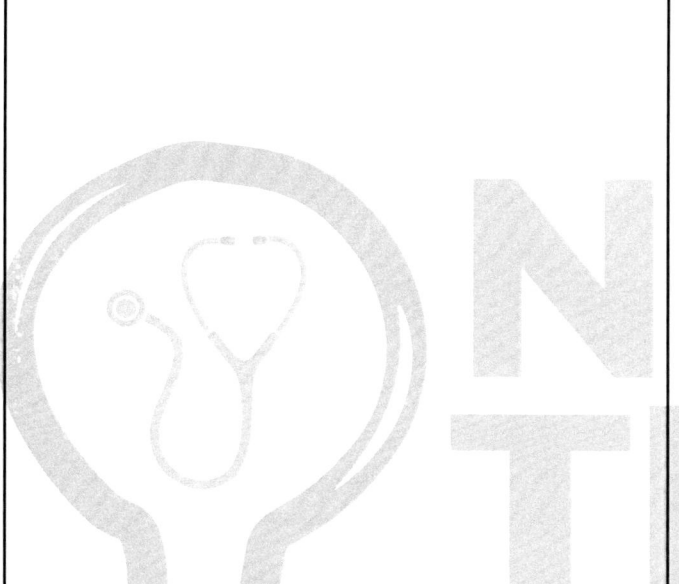

Priority Assessments or Cues

1

2

3

Priority Labs & Diagnostics

1

2

3

Priority Nursing Interventions

1

2

3

Priority Medications

1

2

3

Priority Potential & Actual Complications

1

2

3

Priority Collaborative Goals

1

2

3

NurseThink® Quick

NEXT GEN LEARNING – NCLEX® TEST PLAN

Safe and Effective Care: Management of Care, Coordinated Care, Safety and Infection Control

Health Promotion and Maintenance

Psychosocial Integrity

Physiological Integrity: Basic Care and Comfort, Pharmacological and Parenteral Therapies, Reduction of Risk Potential, and Physiological Adaptation

QUALITY AND SAFETY COMPETENCIES

Patient-Centered Care

Teamwork and Collaboration

Evidence-Based Practice

Quality Improvement

Safety

Informatics

Peer Review: _____   Faculty Review: _____

Grade Tracker

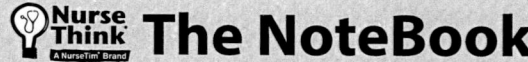
Related Concepts	Related Exemplars/Diseases

Reading/Resources - Clinical Judgment	Class/Lab/Clinical – Clinical Judgment

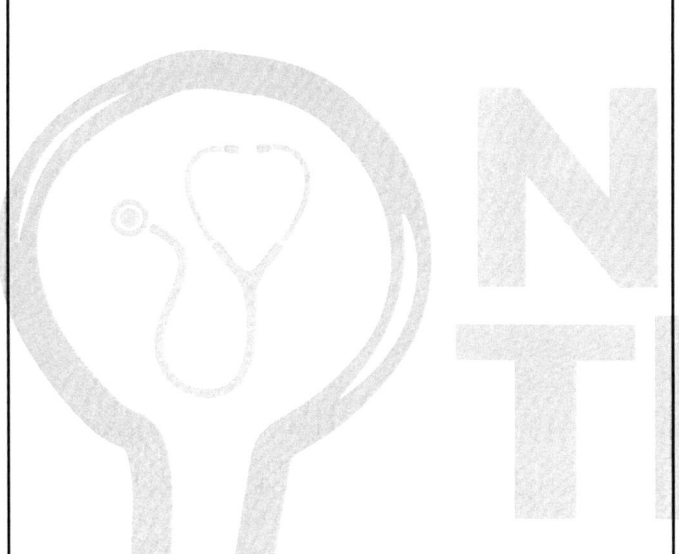

Priority Assessments or Cues	Priority Labs & Diagnostics	Priority Nursing Interventions
1	1	1
2	2	2
3	3	3

Priority Medications	Priority Potential & Actual Complications	Priority Collaborative Goals
1	1	1
2	2	2
3	3	3

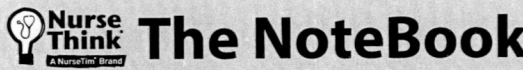
NurseThink® Quick

NEXT GEN LEARNING – NCLEX® TEST PLAN

Safe and Effective Care: Management of Care, Coordinated Care, Safety and Infection Control

Health Promotion and Maintenance

Psychosocial Integrity

Physiological Integrity: Basic Care and Comfort, Pharmacological and Parenteral Therapies, Reduction of Risk Potential, and Physiological Adaptation

QUALITY AND SAFETY COMPETENCIES

Patient-Centered Care

Teamwork and Collaboration

Evidence-Based Practice

Quality Improvement

Safety

Informatics

Peer Review: _____　　　Faculty Review: _____

Grade Tracker

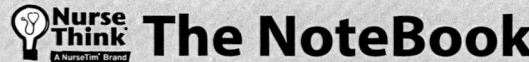
Related Concepts	**Related Exemplars/Diseases**

Reading/Resources - Clinical Judgment	**Class/Lab/Clinical – Clinical Judgment**

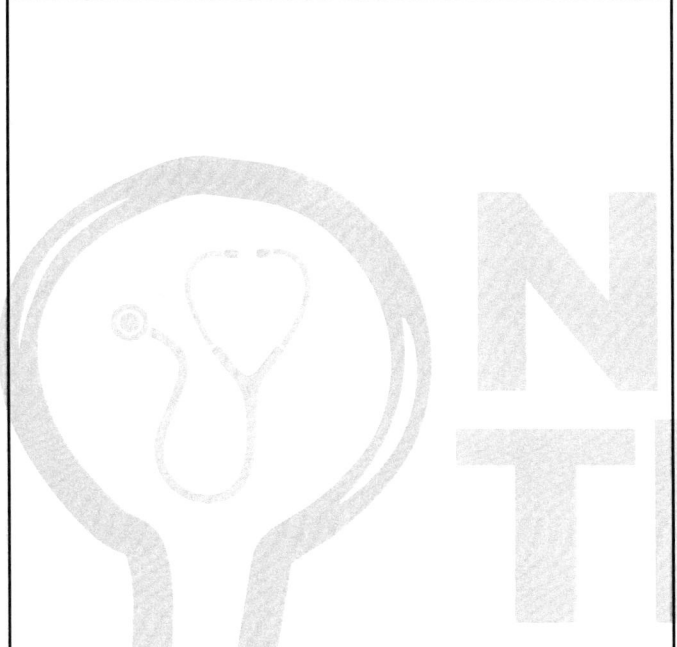

Priority Assessments or Cues

1

2

3

Priority Labs & Diagnostics

1

2

3

Priority Nursing Interventions

1

2

3

Priority Medications

1

2

3

Priority Potential & Actual Complications

1

2

3

Priority Collaborative Goals

1

2

3

NurseThink® Quick

NEXT GEN LEARNING – NCLEX® TEST PLAN

Safe and Effective Care: Management of Care, Coordinated Care, Safety and Infection Control

Health Promotion and Maintenance

Psychosocial Integrity

Physiological Integrity: Basic Care and Comfort, Pharmacological and Parenteral Therapies, Reduction of Risk Potential, and Physiological Adaptation

QUALITY AND SAFETY COMPETENCIES

Patient-Centered Care

Teamwork and Collaboration

Evidence-Based Practice

Quality Improvement

Safety

Informatics

Peer Review: _____   Faculty Review: _____

Grade Tracker

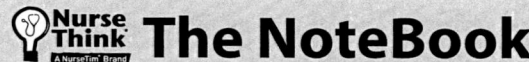
Related Concepts

Related Exemplars/Diseases

Reading/Resources - Clinical Judgment

Class/Lab/Clinical – Clinical Judgment

Priority Assessments or Cues

1

2

3

Priority Labs & Diagnostics

1

2

3

Priority Nursing Interventions

1

2

3

Priority Medications

1

2

3

Priority Potential & Actual Complications

1

2

3

Priority Collaborative Goals

1

2

3

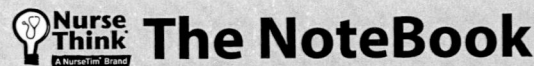
NurseThink® Quick

<table>
<tr><td></td><td></td><td></td></tr>
</table>

NEXT GEN LEARNING – NCLEX® TEST PLAN

Safe and Effective Care: Management of Care, Coordinated Care, Safety and Infection Control

Health Promotion and Maintenance

Psychosocial Integrity

Physiological Integrity: Basic Care and Comfort, Pharmacological and Parenteral Therapies, Reduction of Risk Potential, and Physiological Adaptation

QUALITY AND SAFETY COMPETENCIES

Patient-Centered Care

Teamwork and Collaboration

Evidence-Based Practice

Quality Improvement

Safety

Informatics

Peer Review: _____   Faculty Review: _____

Grade Tracker

<table>
<tr><td></td><td></td><td></td><td></td><td></td><td></td><td></td><td></td><td></td><td></td><td></td><td></td><td></td><td></td><td></td></tr>
</table>

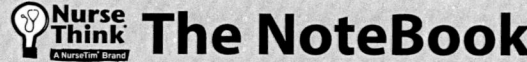
Related Concepts

Related Exemplars/Diseases

Reading/Resources - Clinical Judgment

Class/Lab/Clinical – Clinical Judgment

Priority Assessments or Cues

1

2

3

Priority Labs & Diagnostics

1

2

3

Priority Nursing Interventions

1

2

3

Priority Medications

1

2

3

Priority Potential & Actual Complications

1

2

3

Priority Collaborative Goals

1

2

3

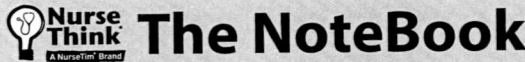
NurseThink® Quick

NEXT GEN LEARNING – NCLEX® TEST PLAN

Safe and Effective Care: Management of Care, Coordinated Care, Safety and Infection Control

Health Promotion and Maintenance

Psychosocial Integrity

Physiological Integrity: Basic Care and Comfort, Pharmacological and Parenteral Therapies, Reduction of Risk Potential, and Physiological Adaptation

QUALITY AND SAFETY COMPETENCIES

Patient-Centered Care

Teamwork and Collaboration

Evidence-Based Practice

Quality Improvement

Safety

Informatics

Peer Review: _____   Faculty Review: _____

Grade Tracker

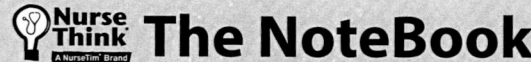
Related Concepts	Related Exemplars/Diseases

Reading/Resources - Clinical Judgment	Class/Lab/Clinical – Clinical Judgment

Priority Assessments or Cues
1
2
3

Priority Labs & Diagnostics
1
2
3

Priority Nursing Interventions
1
2
3

Priority Medications
1
2
3

Priority Potential & Actual Complications
1
2
3

Priority Collaborative Goals
1
2
3

NurseThink® Quick

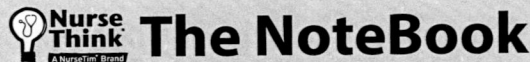

NEXT GEN LEARNING – NCLEX® TEST PLAN

Safe and Effective Care: Management of Care, Coordinated Care, Safety and Infection Control

Health Promotion and Maintenance

Psychosocial Integrity

Physiological Integrity: Basic Care and Comfort, Pharmacological and Parenteral Therapies, Reduction of Risk Potential, and Physiological Adaptation

QUALITY AND SAFETY COMPETENCIES

Patient-Centered Care

Teamwork and Collaboration

Evidence-Based Practice

Quality Improvement

Safety

Informatics

Peer Review: _____   Faculty Review: _____

Grade Tracker

Related Concepts	Related Exemplars/Diseases

Reading/Resources - Clinical Judgment	Class/Lab/Clinical – Clinical Judgment

Priority Assessments or Cues	Priority Labs & Diagnostics	Priority Nursing Interventions
1	1	1
2	2	2
3	3	3

Priority Medications	Priority Potential & Actual Complications	Priority Collaborative Goals
1	1	1
2	2	2
3	3	3

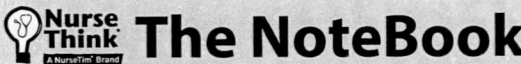
NurseThink® Quick

NEXT GEN LEARNING – NCLEX® TEST PLAN

Safe and Effective Care: Management of Care, Coordinated Care, Safety and Infection Control

Health Promotion and Maintenance

Psychosocial Integrity

Physiological Integrity: Basic Care and Comfort, Pharmacological and Parenteral Therapies, Reduction of Risk Potential, and Physiological Adaptation

QUALITY AND SAFETY COMPETENCIES

Patient-Centered Care

Teamwork and Collaboration

Evidence-Based Practice

Quality Improvement

Safety

Informatics

Peer Review: _____   Faculty Review: _____

Grade Tracker

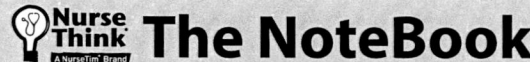

Related Concepts

Related Exemplars/Diseases

Reading/Resources - Clinical Judgment

Class/Lab/Clinical – Clinical Judgment

Priority Assessments or Cues

1
2
3

Priority Labs & Diagnostics

1
2
3

Priority Nursing Interventions

1
2
3

Priority Medications

1
2
3

Priority Potential & Actual Complications

1
2
3

Priority Collaborative Goals

1
2
3

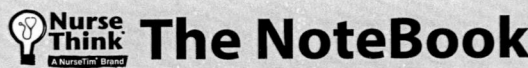
NurseThink® Quick

NEXT GEN LEARNING – NCLEX® TEST PLAN

Safe and Effective Care: Management of Care, Coordinated Care, Safety and Infection Control

Health Promotion and Maintenance

Psychosocial Integrity

Physiological Integrity: Basic Care and Comfort, Pharmacological and Parenteral Therapies, Reduction of Risk Potential, and Physiological Adaptation

QUALITY AND SAFETY COMPETENCIES

Patient-Centered Care

Teamwork and Collaboration

Evidence-Based Practice

Quality Improvement

Safety

Informatics

Peer Review: _____ Faculty Review: _____

Grade Tracker

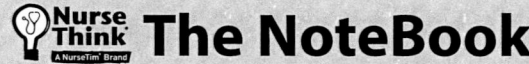

Related Concepts	**Related Exemplars/Diseases**

Reading/Resources - Clinical Judgment	**Class/Lab/Clinical – Clinical Judgment**
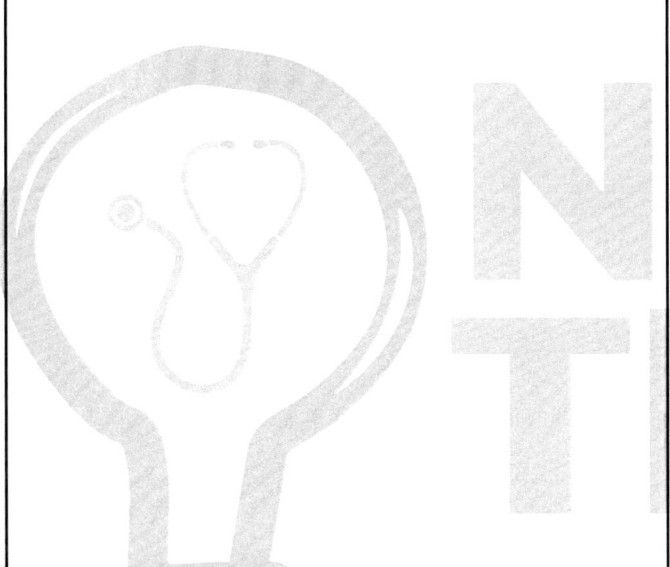	

Priority Assessments or Cues	**Priority Labs & Diagnostics**	**Priority Nursing Interventions**
1	1	1
2	2	2
3	3	3

Priority Medications	**Priority Potential & Actual Complications**	**Priority Collaborative Goals**
1	1	1
2	2	2
3	3	3

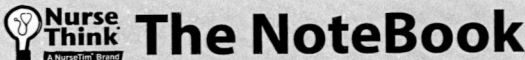
NurseThink® Quick

NEXT GEN LEARNING – NCLEX® TEST PLAN

Safe and Effective Care: Management of Care, Coordinated Care, Safety and Infection Control

Health Promotion and Maintenance

Psychosocial Integrity

Physiological Integrity: Basic Care and Comfort, Pharmacological and Parenteral Therapies, Reduction of Risk Potential, and Physiological Adaptation

QUALITY AND SAFETY COMPETENCIES

Patient-Centered Care

Teamwork and Collaboration

Evidence-Based Practice

Quality Improvement

Safety

Informatics

Peer Review: _____   Faculty Review: _____

Grade Tracker

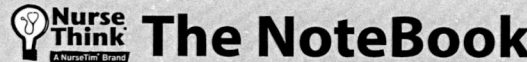
Related Concepts

Related Exemplars/Diseases

Reading/Resources - Clinical Judgment

Class/Lab/Clinical – Clinical Judgment

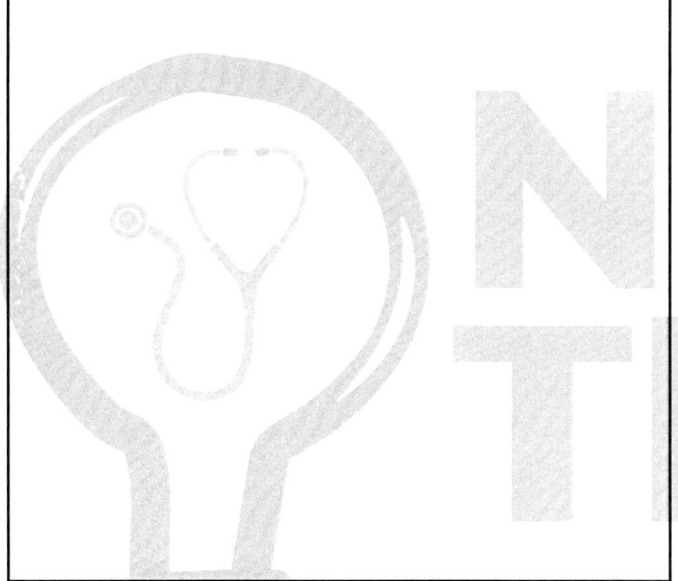

Priority Assessments or Cues

1

2

3

Priority Labs & Diagnostics

1

2

3

Priority Nursing Interventions

1

2

3

Priority Medications

1

2

3

Priority Potential & Actual Complications

1

2

3

Priority Collaborative Goals

1

2

3

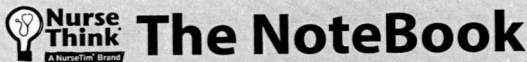
NurseThink® Quick

NEXT GEN LEARNING – NCLEX® TEST PLAN

Safe and Effective Care: Management of Care, Coordinated Care, Safety and Infection Control

Health Promotion and Maintenance

Psychosocial Integrity

Physiological Integrity: Basic Care and Comfort, Pharmacological and Parenteral Therapies, Reduction of Risk Potential, and Physiological Adaptation

QUALITY AND SAFETY COMPETENCIES

Patient-Centered Care

Teamwork and Collaboration

Evidence-Based Practice

Quality Improvement

Safety

Informatics

Peer Review: _____   Faculty Review: _____

Grade Tracker

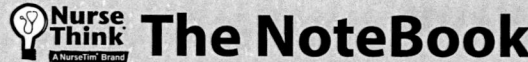
Related Concepts

Related Exemplars/Diseases

Reading/Resources - Clinical Judgment

Class/Lab/Clinical – Clinical Judgment

Priority Assessments or Cues

1

2

3

Priority Labs & Diagnostics

1

2

3

Priority Nursing Interventions

1

2

3

Priority Medications

1

2

3

Priority Potential & Actual Complications

1

2

3

Priority Collaborative Goals

1

2

3

NurseThink® Quick

NEXT GEN LEARNING – NCLEX® TEST PLAN

Safe and Effective Care: Management of Care, Coordinated Care, Safety and Infection Control

Health Promotion and Maintenance

Psychosocial Integrity

Physiological Integrity: Basic Care and Comfort, Pharmacological and Parenteral Therapies, Reduction of Risk Potential, and Physiological Adaptation

QUALITY AND SAFETY COMPETENCIES

Patient-Centered Care

Teamwork and Collaboration

Evidence-Based Practice

Quality Improvement

Safety

Informatics

Peer Review: _____   Faculty Review: _____

Grade Tracker

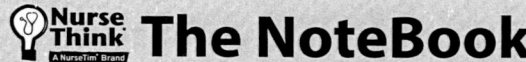
Related Concepts	**Related Exemplars/Diseases**

Reading/Resources - Clinical Judgment	**Class/Lab/Clinical – Clinical Judgment**

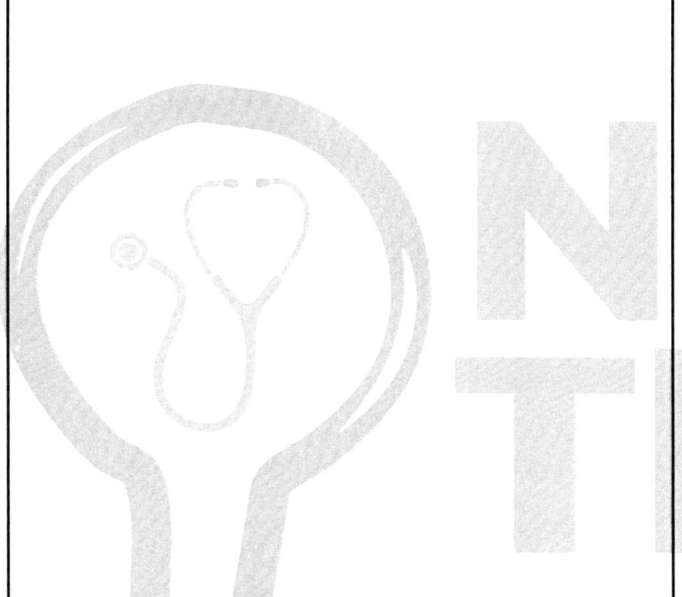

Priority Assessments or Cues	**Priority Labs & Diagnostics**	**Priority Nursing Interventions**
1	1	1
2	2	2
3	3	3

Priority Medications	**Priority Potential & Actual Complications**	**Priority Collaborative Goals**
1	1	1
2	2	2
3	3	3

NurseThink® Quick

NEXT GEN LEARNING – NCLEX® TEST PLAN

Safe and Effective Care: Management of Care, Coordinated Care, Safety and Infection Control

Health Promotion and Maintenance

Psychosocial Integrity

Physiological Integrity: Basic Care and Comfort, Pharmacological and Parenteral Therapies, Reduction of Risk Potential, and Physiological Adaptation

QUALITY AND SAFETY COMPETENCIES

Patient-Centered Care

Teamwork and Collaboration

Evidence-Based Practice

Quality Improvement

Safety

Informatics

Peer Review: _____   Faculty Review: _____

Grade Tracker

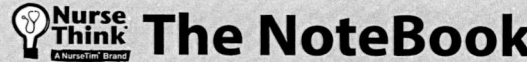

Related Concepts

Related Exemplars/Diseases

Reading/Resources - Clinical Judgment

Class/Lab/Clinical – Clinical Judgment

Priority Assessments or Cues

1

2

3

Priority Labs & Diagnostics

1

2

3

Priority Nursing Interventions

1

2

3

Priority Medications

1

2

3

Priority Potential & Actual Complications

1

2

3

Priority Collaborative Goals

1

2

3

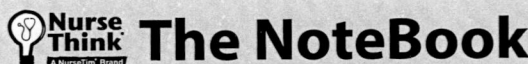
NurseThink® Quick

NEXT GEN LEARNING – NCLEX® TEST PLAN

Safe and Effective Care: Management of Care, Coordinated Care, Safety and Infection Control

Health Promotion and Maintenance

Psychosocial Integrity

Physiological Integrity: Basic Care and Comfort, Pharmacological and Parenteral Therapies, Reduction of Risk Potential, and Physiological Adaptation

QUALITY AND SAFETY COMPETENCIES

Patient-Centered Care

Teamwork and Collaboration

Evidence-Based Practice

Quality Improvement

Safety

Informatics

Peer Review: _____   Faculty Review: _____

Grade Tracker

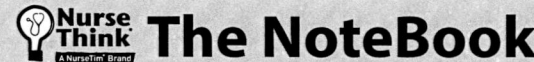
Related Concepts	**Related Exemplars/Diseases**

Reading/Resources - Clinical Judgment	**Class/Lab/Clinical – Clinical Judgment**

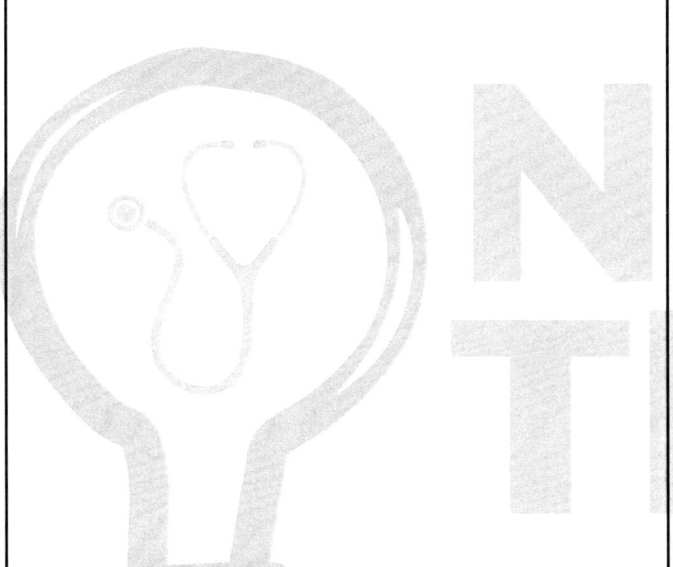

Priority Assessments or Cues

1

2

3

Priority Labs & Diagnostics

1

2

3

Priority Nursing Interventions

1

2

3

Priority Medications

1

2

3

Priority Potential & Actual Complications

1

2

3

Priority Collaborative Goals

1

2

3

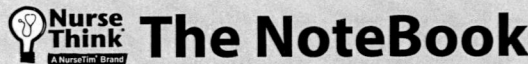
NurseThink® Quick

NEXT GEN LEARNING – NCLEX® TEST PLAN

Safe and Effective Care: Management of Care, Coordinated Care, Safety and Infection Control

Health Promotion and Maintenance

Psychosocial Integrity

Physiological Integrity: Basic Care and Comfort, Pharmacological and Parenteral Therapies, Reduction of Risk Potential, and Physiological Adaptation

QUALITY AND SAFETY COMPETENCIES

Patient-Centered Care

Teamwork and Collaboration

Evidence-Based Practice

Quality Improvement

Safety

Informatics

Peer Review: _____   Faculty Review: _____

Grade Tracker

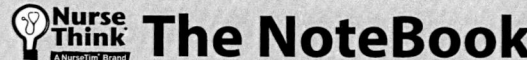
Related Concepts	**Related Exemplars/Diseases**

Reading/Resources - Clinical Judgment	**Class/Lab/Clinical – Clinical Judgment**

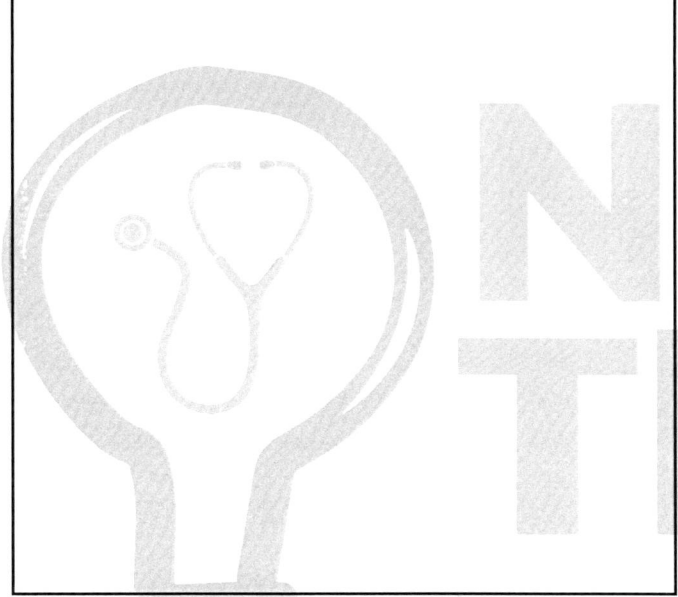

Priority Assessments or Cues	**Priority Labs & Diagnostics**	**Priority Nursing Interventions**
1	1	1
2	2	2
3	3	3

Priority Medications	**Priority Potential & Actual Complications**	**Priority Collaborative Goals**
1	1	1
2	2	2
3	3	3

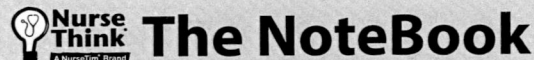
NurseThink® Quick

Choose the related National Patient Safety Goals (NPSG) (www.jointcommission.org)	Priority Pre and Post-Procedure Assessment	

NEXT GEN LEARNING – NCLEX® TEST PLAN

Safe and Effective Care: Management of Care, Coordinated Care, Safety and Infection Control

Health Promotion and Maintenance

Psychosocial Integrity

Physiological Integrity: Basic Care and Comfort, Pharmacological and Parenteral Therapies, Reduction of Risk Potential, and Physiological Adaptation

QUALITY AND SAFETY COMPETENCIES

Patient-Centered Care

Teamwork and Collaboration

Evidence-Based Practice

Quality Improvement

Safety

Informatics

Peer Review: _____ Faculty Review: _____

Grade Tracker

Related Concepts

Related Exemplars/Diseases

Reading/Resources - Clinical Judgment

Class/Lab/Clinical – Clinical Judgment

Priority Assessments or Cues
1
2
3

Priority Labs & Diagnostics
1
2
3

Priority Nursing Interventions
1
2
3

Priority Medications
1
2
3

Priority Potential & Actual Complications
1
2
3

Priority Collaborative Goals
1
2
3

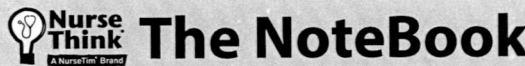

NurseThink® Quick

Choose the related National Patient Safety Goals (NPSG) (www.jointcommission.org)	Priority Pre and Post-Procedure Assessment	

NEXT GEN LEARNING – NCLEX® TEST PLAN

Safe and Effective Care: Management of Care, Coordinated Care, Safety and Infection Control

Health Promotion and Maintenance

Psychosocial Integrity

Physiological Integrity: Basic Care and Comfort, Pharmacological and Parenteral Therapies, Reduction of Risk Potential, and Physiological Adaptation

QUALITY AND SAFETY COMPETENCIES

Patient-Centered Care

Teamwork and Collaboration

Evidence-Based Practice

Quality Improvement

Safety

Informatics

Peer Review: _____　　Faculty Review: _____

Grade Tracker

Related Concepts

Related Exemplars/Diseases

Reading/Resources - Clinical Judgment

Class/Lab/Clinical – Clinical Judgment

Priority Assessments or Cues

1

2

3

Priority Labs & Diagnostics

1

2

3

Priority Nursing Interventions

1

2

3

Priority Medications

1

2

3

Priority Potential & Actual Complications

1

2

3

Priority Collaborative Goals

1

2

3

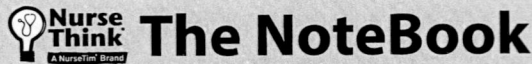

NurseThink® Quick

Choose the related National Patient Safety Goals (NPSG) (www.jointcommission.org)	Priority Pre and Post-Procedure Assessment	

NEXT GEN LEARNING – NCLEX® TEST PLAN

Safe and Effective Care: Management of Care, Coordinated Care, Safety and Infection Control

Health Promotion and Maintenance

Psychosocial Integrity

Physiological Integrity: Basic Care and Comfort, Pharmacological and Parenteral Therapies, Reduction of Risk Potential, and Physiological Adaptation

QUALITY AND SAFETY COMPETENCIES

Patient-Centered Care

Teamwork and Collaboration

Evidence-Based Practice

Quality Improvement

Safety

Informatics

Peer Review: _____   Faculty Review: _____

Grade Tracker

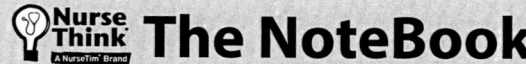
Related Concepts	Related Exemplars/Diseases

Reading/Resources - Clinical Judgment	Class/Lab/Clinical – Clinical Judgment
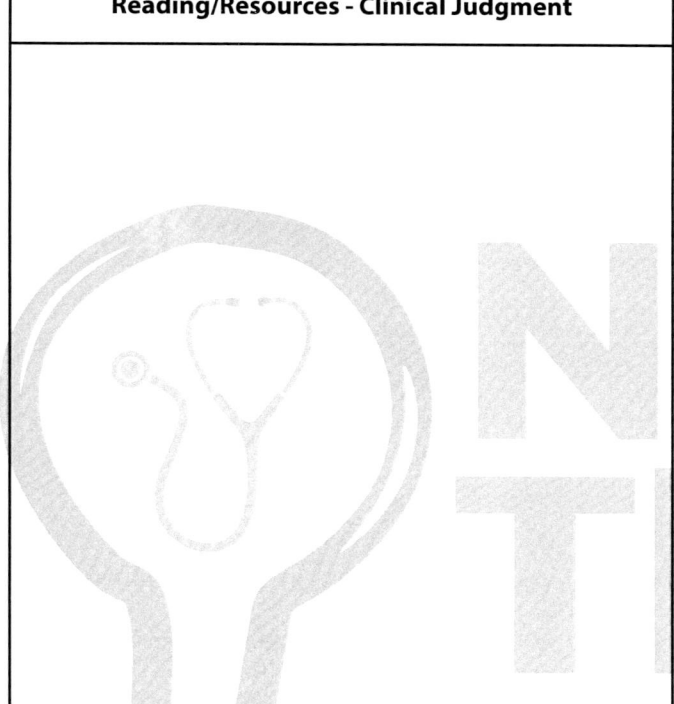	

Priority Assessments or Cues

1

2

3

Priority Labs & Diagnostics

1

2

3

Priority Nursing Interventions

1

2

3

Priority Medications

1

2

3

Priority Potential & Actual Complications

1

2

3

Priority Collaborative Goals

1

2

3

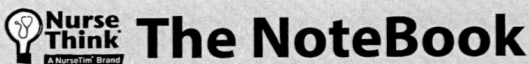
NurseThink® Quick

Choose the related National Patient Safety Goals (NPSG) (www.jointcommission.org)	Priority Pre and Post-Procedure Assessment	

NEXT GEN LEARNING – NCLEX® TEST PLAN

Safe and Effective Care: Management of Care, Coordinated Care, Safety and Infection Control

Health Promotion and Maintenance

Psychosocial Integrity

Physiological Integrity: Basic Care and Comfort, Pharmacological and Parenteral Therapies, Reduction of Risk Potential, and Physiological Adaptation

QUALITY AND SAFETY COMPETENCIES

Patient-Centered Care

Teamwork and Collaboration

Evidence-Based Practice

Quality Improvement

Safety

Informatics

Peer Review: _____   Faculty Review: _____

Grade Tracker

Related Concepts

Related Exemplars/Diseases

Reading/Resources - Clinical Judgment

Class/Lab/Clinical – Clinical Judgment

Priority Assessments or Cues

1
2
3

Priority Labs & Diagnostics

1
2
3

Priority Nursing Interventions

1
2
3

Priority Medications

1
2
3

Priority Potential & Actual Complications

1
2
3

Priority Collaborative Goals

1
2
3

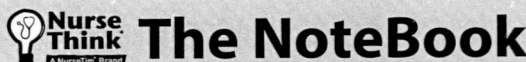
NurseThink® Quick

Choose the related National Patient Safety Goals (NPSG) (www.jointcommission.org)	Priority Pre and Post-Procedure Assessment	

NEXT GEN LEARNING – NCLEX® TEST PLAN

Safe and Effective Care: Management of Care, Coordinated Care, Safety and Infection Control

Health Promotion and Maintenance

Psychosocial Integrity

Physiological Integrity: Basic Care and Comfort, Pharmacological and Parenteral Therapies, Reduction of Risk Potential, and Physiological Adaptation

QUALITY AND SAFETY COMPETENCIES

Patient-Centered Care

Teamwork and Collaboration

Evidence-Based Practice

Quality Improvement

Safety

Informatics

Peer Review: _____   Faculty Review: _____

Grade Tracker

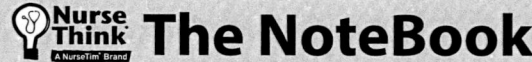
Related Concepts

Related Exemplars/Diseases

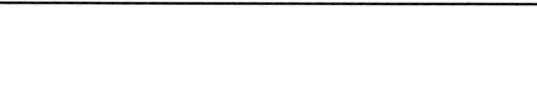

Reading/Resources - Clinical Judgment

Class/Lab/Clinical – Clinical Judgment

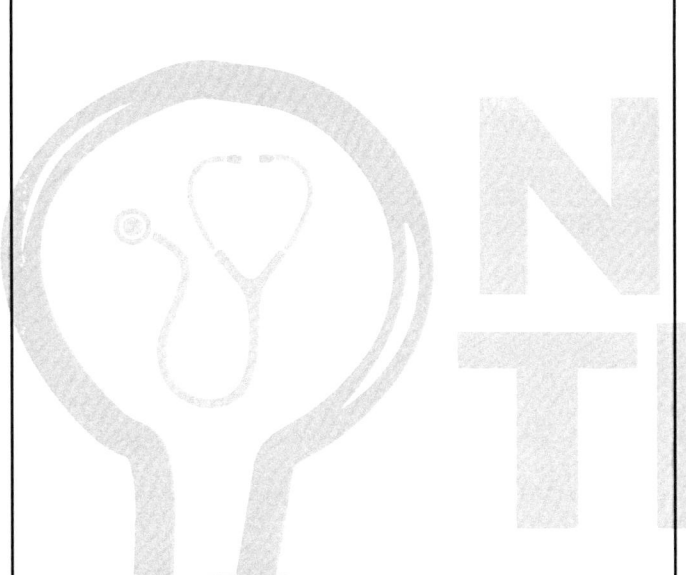

Priority Assessments or Cues

1

2

3

Priority Labs & Diagnostics

1

2

3

Priority Nursing Interventions

1

2

3

Priority Medications

1

2

3

Priority Potential & Actual Complications

1

2

3

Priority Collaborative Goals

1

2

3

NurseThink® Quick

Choose the related National Patient Safety Goals (NPSG) (www.jointcommission.org)	Priority Pre and Post-Procedure Assessment	

NEXT GEN LEARNING – NCLEX® TEST PLAN

Safe and Effective Care: Management of Care, Coordinated Care, Safety and Infection Control

Health Promotion and Maintenance

Psychosocial Integrity

Physiological Integrity: Basic Care and Comfort, Pharmacological and Parenteral Therapies, Reduction of Risk Potential, and Physiological Adaptation

QUALITY AND SAFETY COMPETENCIES

Patient-Centered Care

Teamwork and Collaboration

Evidence-Based Practice

Quality Improvement

Safety

Informatics

Peer Review: _____   Faculty Review: _____

Grade Tracker

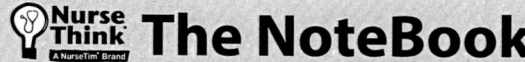
Related Concepts	Related Exemplars/Diseases

Reading/Resources - Clinical Judgment	Class/Lab/Clinical – Clinical Judgment

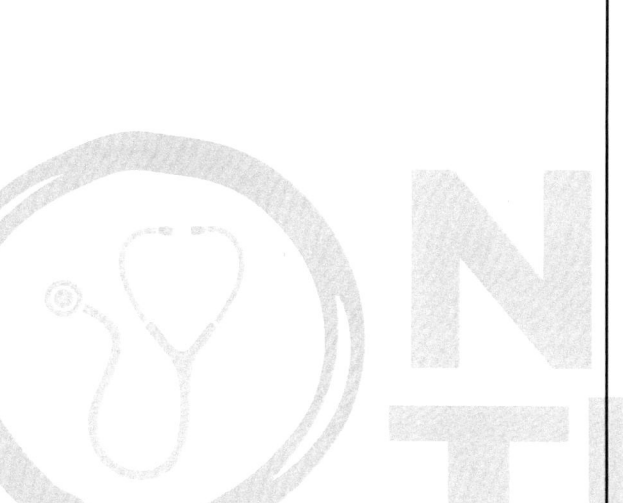

Priority Assessments or Cues	Priority Labs & Diagnostics	Priority Nursing Interventions
1	1	1
2	2	2
3	3	3

Priority Medications	Priority Potential & Actual Complications	Priority Collaborative Goals
1	1	1
2	2	2
3	3	3

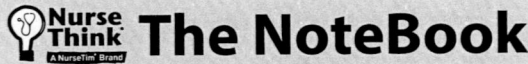
NurseThink® Quick

Choose the related National Patient Safety Goals (NPSG) (www.jointcommission.org)	Priority Pre and Post-Procedure Assessment	

NEXT GEN LEARNING – NCLEX® TEST PLAN

Safe and Effective Care: Management of Care, Coordinated Care, Safety and Infection Control

Health Promotion and Maintenance

Psychosocial Integrity

Physiological Integrity: Basic Care and Comfort, Pharmacological and Parenteral Therapies, Reduction of Risk Potential, and Physiological Adaptation

QUALITY AND SAFETY COMPETENCIES

Patient-Centered Care

Teamwork and Collaboration

Evidence-Based Practice

Quality Improvement

Safety

Informatics

Peer Review: _____   Faculty Review: _____

Grade Tracker

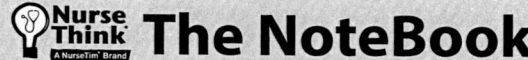
Related Concepts	Related Exemplars/Diseases

Reading/Resources - Clinical Judgment	Class/Lab/Clinical – Clinical Judgment
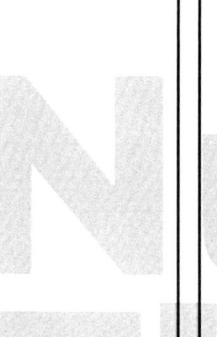	

Priority Assessments or Cues	Priority Labs & Diagnostics	Priority Nursing Interventions
1	1	1
2	2	2
3	3	3

Priority Medications	Priority Potential & Actual Complications	Priority Collaborative Goals
1	1	1
2	2	2
3	3	3

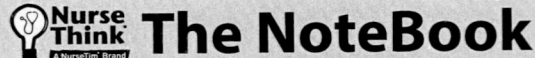
NurseThink® Quick

Choose the related National Patient Safety Goals (NPSG) (www.jointcommission.org)	Priority Pre and Post-Procedure Assessment	

NEXT GEN LEARNING – NCLEX® TEST PLAN

Safe and Effective Care: Management of Care, Coordinated Care, Safety and Infection Control

Health Promotion and Maintenance

Psychosocial Integrity

Physiological Integrity: Basic Care and Comfort, Pharmacological and Parenteral Therapies, Reduction of Risk Potential, and Physiological Adaptation

QUALITY AND SAFETY COMPETENCIES

Patient-Centered Care

Teamwork and Collaboration

Evidence-Based Practice

Quality Improvement

Safety

Informatics

Peer Review: _____   Faculty Review: _____

Grade Tracker

Related Concepts	Related Exemplars/Diseases

Reading/Resources - Clinical Judgment	Class/Lab/Clinical – Clinical Judgment

Priority Assessments or Cues	Priority Labs & Diagnostics	Priority Nursing Interventions
1	1	1
2	2	2
3	3	3

Priority Medications	Priority Potential & Actual Complications	Priority Collaborative Goals
1	1	1
2	2	2
3	3	3

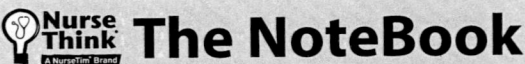

NurseThink® Quick

Choose the related National Patient Safety Goals (NPSG) (www.jointcommission.org)	Priority Pre and Post-Procedure Assessment	

NEXT GEN LEARNING – NCLEX® TEST PLAN

Safe and Effective Care: Management of Care, Coordinated Care, Safety and Infection Control

Health Promotion and Maintenance

Psychosocial Integrity

Physiological Integrity: Basic Care and Comfort, Pharmacological and Parenteral Therapies, Reduction of Risk Potential, and Physiological Adaptation

QUALITY AND SAFETY COMPETENCIES

Patient-Centered Care

Teamwork and Collaboration

Evidence-Based Practice

Quality Improvement

Safety

Informatics

Peer Review: _____   Faculty Review: _____

Grade Tracker

Related Concepts

Related Exemplars/Diseases

Reading/Resources - Clinical Judgment

Class/Lab/Clinical – Clinical Judgment

Priority Assessments or Cues
1
2
3

Priority Labs & Diagnostics
1
2
3

Priority Nursing Interventions
1
2
3

Priority Medications
1
2
3

Priority Potential & Actual Complications
1
2
3

Priority Collaborative Goals
1
2
3

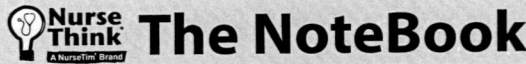
NurseThink® Quick

Choose the related National Patient Safety Goals (NPSG) (www.jointcommission.org)	Priority Pre and Post-Procedure Assessment	

NEXT GEN LEARNING – NCLEX® TEST PLAN

Safe and Effective Care: Management of Care, Coordinated Care, Safety and Infection Control

Health Promotion and Maintenance

Psychosocial Integrity

Physiological Integrity: Basic Care and Comfort, Pharmacological and Parenteral Therapies, Reduction of Risk Potential, and Physiological Adaptation

QUALITY AND SAFETY COMPETENCIES

Patient-Centered Care

Teamwork and Collaboration

Evidence-Based Practice

Quality Improvement

Safety

Informatics

Peer Review: _____ Faculty Review: _____

Grade Tracker

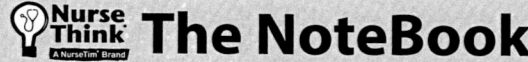
Related Concepts	**Related Exemplars/Diseases**

Reading/Resources - Clinical Judgment	**Class/Lab/Clinical – Clinical Judgment**

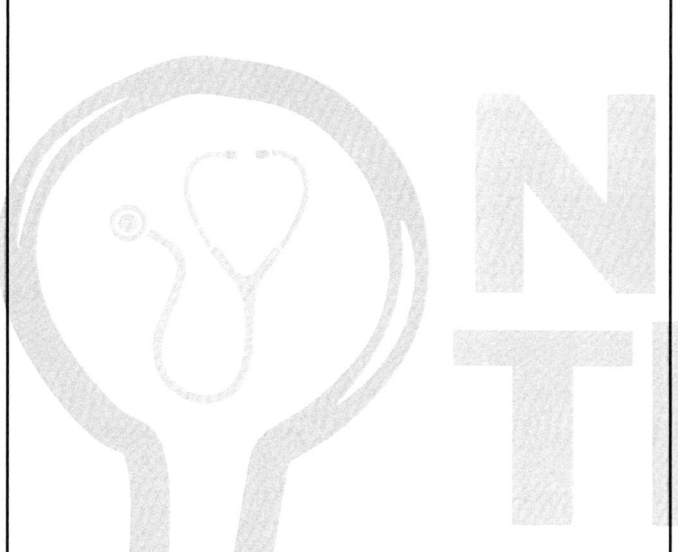

Priority Assessments or Cues	**Priority Labs & Diagnostics**	**Priority Nursing Interventions**
1	1	1
2	2	2
3	3	3

Priority Medications	**Priority Potential & Actual Complications**	**Priority Collaborative Goals**
1	1	1
2	2	2
3	3	3

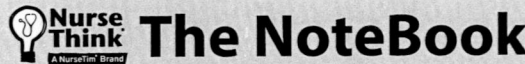
NurseThink® Quick

Choose the related National Patient Safety Goals (NPSG) (www.jointcommission.org)	Priority Pre and Post-Procedure Assessment	

NEXT GEN LEARNING – NCLEX® TEST PLAN

Safe and Effective Care: Management of Care, Coordinated Care, Safety and Infection Control

Health Promotion and Maintenance

Psychosocial Integrity

Physiological Integrity: Basic Care and Comfort, Pharmacological and Parenteral Therapies, Reduction of Risk Potential, and Physiological Adaptation

QUALITY AND SAFETY COMPETENCIES

Patient-Centered Care

Teamwork and Collaboration

Evidence-Based Practice

Quality Improvement

Safety

Informatics

Peer Review: _____   Faculty Review: _____

Grade Tracker

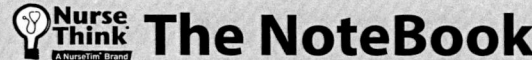

Related Concepts	Related Exemplars/Diseases

Reading/Resources - Clinical Judgment	Class/Lab/Clinical – Clinical Judgment

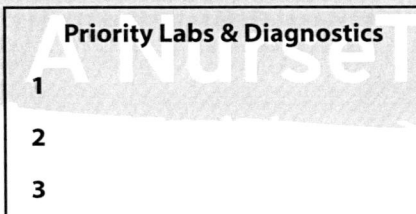

Priority Assessments or Cues	Priority Labs & Diagnostics	Priority Nursing Interventions
1	1	1
2	2	2
3	3	3

Priority Medications	Priority Potential & Actual Complications	Priority Collaborative Goals
1	1	1
2	2	2
3	3	3

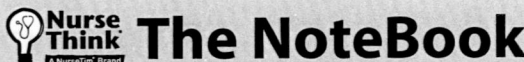
NurseThink® Quick

Choose the related National Patient Safety Goals (NPSG) (www.jointcommission.org)	Priority Pre and Post-Procedure Assessment	

NEXT GEN LEARNING – NCLEX® TEST PLAN

Safe and Effective Care: Management of Care, Coordinated Care, Safety and Infection Control

Health Promotion and Maintenance

Psychosocial Integrity

Physiological Integrity: Basic Care and Comfort, Pharmacological and Parenteral Therapies, Reduction of Risk Potential, and Physiological Adaptation

QUALITY AND SAFETY COMPETENCIES

Patient-Centered Care

Teamwork and Collaboration

Evidence-Based Practice

Quality Improvement

Safety

Informatics

Peer Review: _____   Faculty Review: _____

Grade Tracker

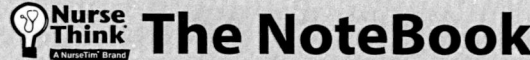

Related Concepts	**Related Exemplars/Diseases**

Reading/Resources - Clinical Judgment	**Class/Lab/Clinical – Clinical Judgment**

Priority Assessments or Cues	**Priority Labs & Diagnostics**	**Priority Nursing Interventions**
1	1	1
2	2	2
3	3	3

Priority Medications	**Priority Potential & Actual Complications**	**Priority Collaborative Goals**
1	1	1
2	2	2
3	3	3

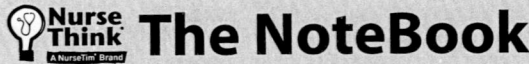
NurseThink® Quick

Choose the related National Patient Safety Goals (NPSG) (www.jointcommission.org)	Priority Pre and Post-Procedure Assessment	

NEXT GEN LEARNING – NCLEX® TEST PLAN

Safe and Effective Care: Management of Care, Coordinated Care, Safety and Infection Control

Health Promotion and Maintenance

Psychosocial Integrity

Physiological Integrity: Basic Care and Comfort, Pharmacological and Parenteral Therapies, Reduction of Risk Potential, and Physiological Adaptation

QUALITY AND SAFETY COMPETENCIES

Patient-Centered Care

Teamwork and Collaboration

Evidence-Based Practice

Quality Improvement

Safety

Informatics

Peer Review: _____ Faculty Review: _____

Grade Tracker

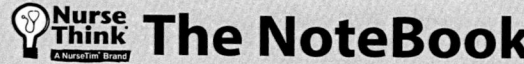
Related Concepts

Related Exemplars/Diseases

Reading/Resources - Clinical Judgment

Class/Lab/Clinical – Clinical Judgment

Priority Assessments or Cues

1

2

3

Priority Labs & Diagnostics

1

2

3

Priority Nursing Interventions

1

2

3

Priority Medications

1

2

3

Priority Potential & Actual Complications

1

2

3

Priority Collaborative Goals

1

2

3

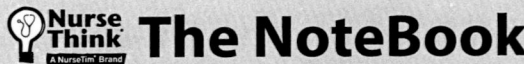
NurseThink® Quick

Choose the related National Patient Safety Goals (NPSG) (www.jointcommission.org)	Priority Pre and Post-Procedure Assessment	

NEXT GEN LEARNING – NCLEX® TEST PLAN

Safe and Effective Care: Management of Care, Coordinated Care, Safety and Infection Control

Health Promotion and Maintenance

Psychosocial Integrity

Physiological Integrity: Basic Care and Comfort, Pharmacological and Parenteral Therapies, Reduction of Risk Potential, and Physiological Adaptation

QUALITY AND SAFETY COMPETENCIES

Patient-Centered Care

Teamwork and Collaboration

Evidence-Based Practice

Quality Improvement

Safety

Informatics

Peer Review: _____   Faculty Review: _____

Grade Tracker

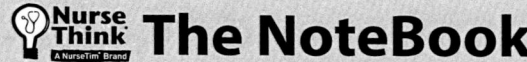

Related Concepts	**Related Exemplars/Diseases**

Reading/Resources - Clinical Judgment	**Class/Lab/Clinical – Clinical Judgment**
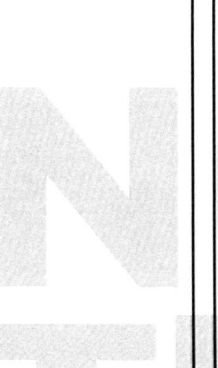	

Priority Assessments or Cues	**Priority Labs & Diagnostics**	**Priority Nursing Interventions**
1	1	1
2	2	2
3	3	3

Priority Medications	**Priority Potential & Actual Complications**	**Priority Collaborative Goals**
1	1	1
2	2	2
3	3	3

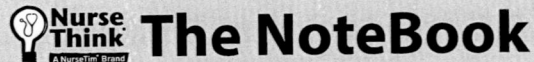
NurseThink® Quick

Choose the related National Patient Safety Goals (NPSG) (www.jointcommission.org)	Priority Pre and Post-Procedure Assessment	

NEXT GEN LEARNING – NCLEX® TEST PLAN

Safe and Effective Care: Management of Care, Coordinated Care, Safety and Infection Control

Health Promotion and Maintenance

Psychosocial Integrity

Physiological Integrity: Basic Care and Comfort, Pharmacological and Parenteral Therapies, Reduction of Risk Potential, and Physiological Adaptation

QUALITY AND SAFETY COMPETENCIES

Patient-Centered Care

Teamwork and Collaboration

Evidence-Based Practice

Quality Improvement

Safety

Informatics

Peer Review: _____   Faculty Review: _____

Grade Tracker

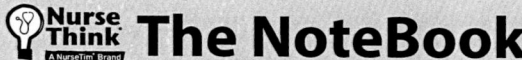
Related Concepts	Related Exemplars/Diseases

Reading/Resources - Clinical Judgment	Class/Lab/Clinical – Clinical Judgment
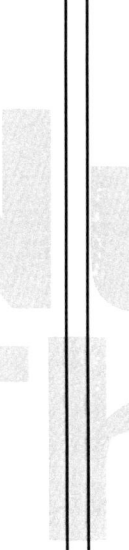	

Priority Assessments or Cues	Priority Labs & Diagnostics	Priority Nursing Interventions
1	1	1
2	2	2
3	3	3

Priority Medications	Priority Potential & Actual Complications	Priority Collaborative Goals
1	1	1
2	2	2
3	3	3

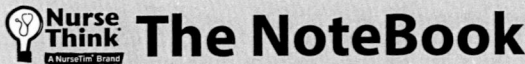
NurseThink® Quick

NEXT GEN LEARNING – NCLEX® TEST PLAN

Safe and Effective Care: Management of Care, Coordinated Care, Safety and Infection Control

Health Promotion and Maintenance

Psychosocial Integrity

Physiological Integrity: Basic Care and Comfort, Pharmacological and Parenteral Therapies, Reduction of Risk Potential, and Physiological Adaptation

QUALITY AND SAFETY COMPETENCIES

Patient-Centered Care

Teamwork and Collaboration

Evidence-Based Practice

Quality Improvement

Safety

Informatics

Peer Review: _____   Faculty Review: _____

Grade Tracker

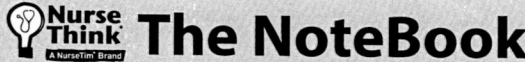

Related Concepts	**Related Exemplars/Diseases**

Reading/Resources - Clinical Judgment	**Class/Lab/Clinical – Clinical Judgment**

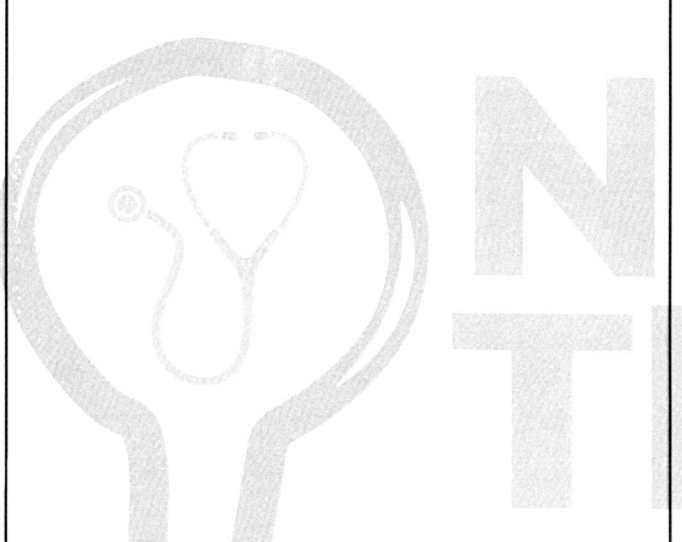

Priority Assessments or Cues	**Priority Labs & Diagnostics**	**Priority Nursing Interventions**
1	1	1
2	2	2
3	3	3

Priority Medications	**Priority Potential & Actual Complications**	**Priority Collaborative Goals**
1	1	1
2	2	2
3	3	3

NurseThink® Quick

NEXT GEN LEARNING – NCLEX® TEST PLAN

Safe and Effective Care: Management of Care, Coordinated Care, Safety and Infection Control

Health Promotion and Maintenance

Psychosocial Integrity

Physiological Integrity: Basic Care and Comfort, Pharmacological and Parenteral Therapies, Reduction of Risk Potential, and Physiological Adaptation

QUALITY AND SAFETY COMPETENCIES

Patient-Centered Care

Teamwork and Collaboration

Evidence-Based Practice

Quality Improvement

Safety

Informatics

Peer Review: _____   Faculty Review: _____

Grade Tracker

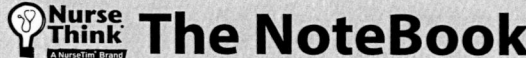
Related Concepts	Related Exemplars/Diseases

Reading/Resources - Clinical Judgment	Class/Lab/Clinical – Clinical Judgment

Priority Assessments or Cues	Priority Labs & Diagnostics	Priority Nursing Interventions
1	1	1
2	2	2
3	3	3

Priority Medications	Priority Potential & Actual Complications	Priority Collaborative Goals
1	1	1
2	2	2
3	3	3

NurseThink® Quick

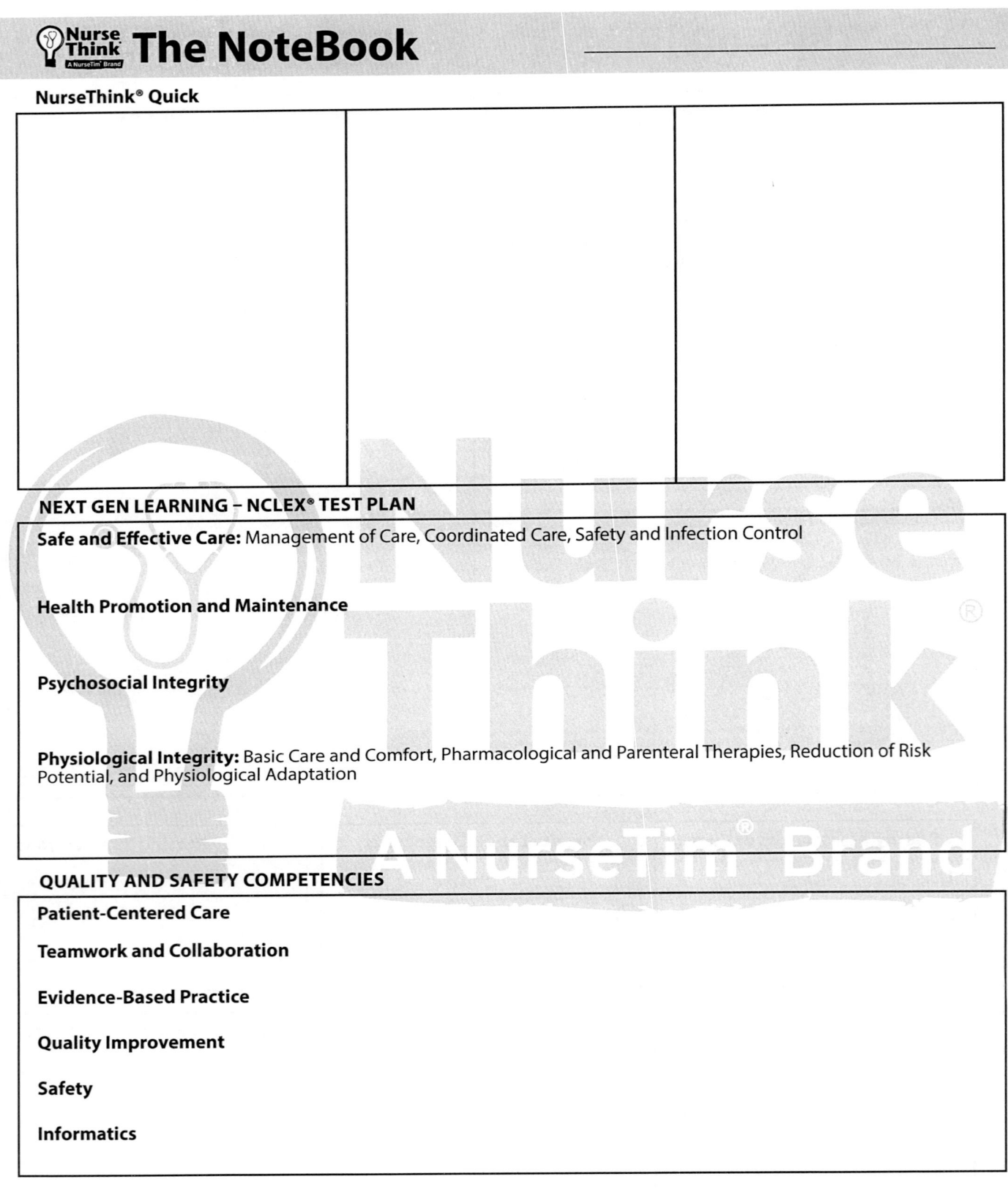

NEXT GEN LEARNING – NCLEX® TEST PLAN

Safe and Effective Care: Management of Care, Coordinated Care, Safety and Infection Control

Health Promotion and Maintenance

Psychosocial Integrity

Physiological Integrity: Basic Care and Comfort, Pharmacological and Parenteral Therapies, Reduction of Risk Potential, and Physiological Adaptation

QUALITY AND SAFETY COMPETENCIES

Patient-Centered Care

Teamwork and Collaboration

Evidence-Based Practice

Quality Improvement

Safety

Informatics

Peer Review: _____   Faculty Review: _____

Grade Tracker

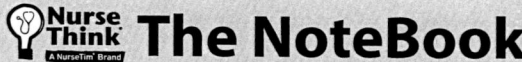
Related Concepts	Related Exemplars/Diseases

Reading/Resources - Clinical Judgment	Class/Lab/Clinical – Clinical Judgment

Priority Assessments or Cues	Priority Labs & Diagnostics	Priority Nursing Interventions
1	1	1
2	2	2
3	3	3

Priority Medications	Priority Potential & Actual Complications	Priority Collaborative Goals
1	1	1
2	2	2
3	3	3

NurseThink® Quick

NEXT GEN LEARNING – NCLEX® TEST PLAN

Safe and Effective Care: Management of Care, Coordinated Care, Safety and Infection Control

Health Promotion and Maintenance

Psychosocial Integrity

Physiological Integrity: Basic Care and Comfort, Pharmacological and Parenteral Therapies, Reduction of Risk Potential, and Physiological Adaptation

QUALITY AND SAFETY COMPETENCIES

Patient-Centered Care

Teamwork and Collaboration

Evidence-Based Practice

Quality Improvement

Safety

Informatics

Peer Review: _____   Faculty Review: _____

Grade Tracker

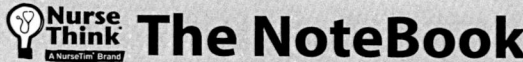

Related Concepts	Related Exemplars/Diseases

Reading/Resources - Clinical Judgment	Class/Lab/Clinical – Clinical Judgment

Priority Assessments or Cues	Priority Labs & Diagnostics	Priority Nursing Interventions
1	1	1
2	2	2
3	3	3

Priority Medications	Priority Potential & Actual Complications	Priority Collaborative Goals
1	1	1
2	2	2
3	3	3

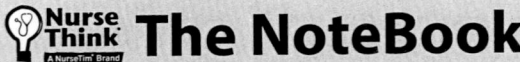

NurseThink® Quick

NEXT GEN LEARNING – NCLEX® TEST PLAN

Safe and Effective Care: Management of Care, Coordinated Care, Safety and Infection Control

Health Promotion and Maintenance

Psychosocial Integrity

Physiological Integrity: Basic Care and Comfort, Pharmacological and Parenteral Therapies, Reduction of Risk Potential, and Physiological Adaptation

QUALITY AND SAFETY COMPETENCIES

Patient-Centered Care

Teamwork and Collaboration

Evidence-Based Practice

Quality Improvement

Safety

Informatics

Peer Review: _____   Faculty Review: _____

Grade Tracker

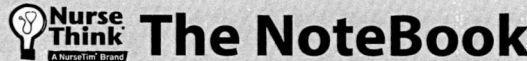
Related Concepts	**Related Exemplars/Diseases**

Reading/Resources - Clinical Judgment	**Class/Lab/Clinical – Clinical Judgment**

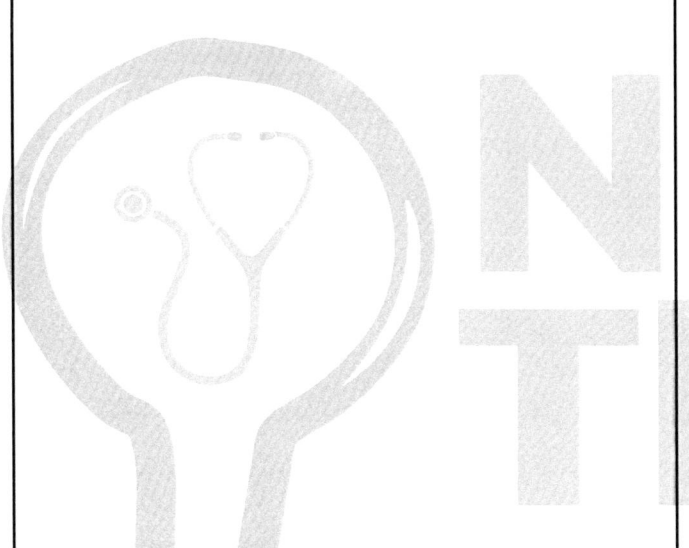

Priority Assessments or Cues	**Priority Labs & Diagnostics**	**Priority Nursing Interventions**
1	1	1
2	2	2
3	3	3

Priority Medications	**Priority Potential & Actual Complications**	**Priority Collaborative Goals**
1	1	1
2	2	2
3	3	3

NurseThink® Quick

NEXT GEN LEARNING – NCLEX® TEST PLAN

Safe and Effective Care: Management of Care, Coordinated Care, Safety and Infection Control

Health Promotion and Maintenance

Psychosocial Integrity

Physiological Integrity: Basic Care and Comfort, Pharmacological and Parenteral Therapies, Reduction of Risk Potential, and Physiological Adaptation

QUALITY AND SAFETY COMPETENCIES

Patient-Centered Care

Teamwork and Collaboration

Evidence-Based Practice

Quality Improvement

Safety

Informatics

Peer Review: _____   Faculty Review: _____

Grade Tracker
